INTERMITTENT FASTING FOR WOMEN

Table of Contents

Introduction

However, there are many differences in regards to how women should follow intermittent fasting. The great news is that women can take part in all the fast's listed in this book, regardless we need to talk about intermittent fasting for women. Then they should have no problem with intermittent fasting, and the problems start to occur when 48 hours+ fasts begin to take place.

Nonetheless, you should know the claims and studies done on women in regards to intermittent fasting. There was one study suggesting that blood sugar worsened in women after three weeks of intermittent fasting. Moreover, many sources are claiming that changes in women menstrual cycle will occur. As we explained before, because of women reproductive system, they are susceptible to lower calories.

Hence, making people believe that women do not indulge in intermittent fasting, which we don't agree. If done tastefully, intermittent fasting has resulted in excellent health and weight loss benefits for women. So in this chapter, we will go thru exactly how intermittent fasting effects women in all aspects, such as hormones, hunger craving, and many more things are on the agenda. With that in mind, let's get into the nitty-gritty.

The key to intermittent fasting for women in autophagy

You might have heard of autophagy in this book so far, now let me explain to you what autophagy truly means. Autophagy is a biological process which comes from the Greek word "auto," meaning "self" and "phagy," meaning "eat." It is a process where our body cleans out the bad cells and replace them with newer healthy ones, which is excellent for anyone looking to live a healthier life.

But sometimes, our body cannot get this process going for hosts of reasons. Manly because we eat the food we can't digest properly, which makes our body work extra hard to cope up with the food instead of getting rid of "bad cells." As we get older, the process becomes less efficient. One of the proven ways to fix this issue, especially for women is by fasting for 12 or more hours and allowing your body to focus more on getting rid of the "bad cells," by replacing them with newer and stronger ones.

This method works exceptionally well, especially on women, to rejuvenate their cells and to see the health benefits. The great news about autophagy is that you don't need to fast for an indefinite amount of time to notice the results, 12 to 16 hours of fast will do. Which means women don't need to put yourself at risk by fasting for a prolonged period; this makes intermittent fasting a tool for women looking to stay young for more extended periods.

Remember that autophagy should not be just for anti-aging purposes, as it can help you with hosts of things. Consider autophagy as a detox for your whole body, and believe it or not most people need it. Forget cleansing diets, and if you truly want to detox your body, then you need to fast for at least 12 hours a day.

For women, 12-16 hours should not result in adverse effects. You will also reduce the risk of cancer because you will have newer and stronger cells at your disposal; another great benefit would be the fact that your metabolism will go up helping you with weight loss.

All in all, promoting the process of autophagy a great way to encourage better health, especially for women. Having healthier cells in a women's body will help you by having a better reproductive system, and you will have a higher chance of conceiving. Even though these claims haven't been backed up, it is still good to know that some excellent benefits come with intermittent fasting for women.

Finally, you will notice benefits such as better skin, better digestion more energy throughout the day. To see the best results, fast for 12 to 16 hours a day, three times a week. Make sure you space out your days, instead of doing all the fasts back to back. If you want to fast through the week as many do, then make sure not to prolong it for more than 6-8 weeks.

Chapter 1 The Skinny on Intermittent Fasting

Intermittent fasting is based on following a particular eating pattern intended to provide optimal health benefits to anyone who embraces it. The pattern requires people to move back and forth between periods of eating and periods of not eating, or fasting. They are timed and scheduled in a very specific manner that is meant to enhance metabolic processes and support individuals in experiencing improved health.

Intermittent fasting itself is less about what to eat and more about when to eat. The most basic variation of the diet actually says nothing about what types of food need to be eaten, though it does encourage eating mindfully and choosing healthy options. Over the years, many adaptations and variations of the diet have been made to support even greater benefits to those who choose to eat this way. Some of these do include specifications on what to eat and when so that you can have even greater benefits from your diet.

When Do You Fast?

Fasting is already a part of your daily life. Every time you go to sleep, you fast for several hours. Then, when you wake up you eat breakfast to break the fast. So, you are essentially already using the intermittent fasting diet as a natural part of your life. When you choose to use this dietary style, you simply adjust your fasting cycle for greater health benefits.

The concept of the intermittent fasting diet is that you simply extend this fasting period and shorten your window of eating. Most commonly, this is done by extending the fasting window to sixteen hours per day and then eating for only eight hours per day.

How long you will fast for and how long you will eat for ultimately depends on what variation of the diet you choose to follow. We will discuss the different adaptations in including how each adaptation is meant to support your health.

Fasting for different lengths of time and eating different amounts of different lengths of time is known to have many health benefits. Typically, you choose the one that has the right considerations for your needs and preferences. Then, you fast for the window of time that is recommended based on that intermittent fasting adaptation.

Why Do You Fast?

The science behind the intermittent fasting diet is based off of the realization that humans have been fasting for many years. Fasting has been used for necessity, religious purposes, and instinctive reasons. Sometimes, when there weren't enough food, humans would fast until there was more. In various religions, fasting is used for various purposes, often as a way to give thanks or show respect to various deities. Instinctively, humans have a tendency to fast when they are feeling sick or stressed out. Fasting is a completely natural practice that humans have been using for thousands of years.

When we refrain from eating for any period of time, various processes in our bodies change. This actually supports our body in thriving during periods of famine or fasting. Most of these changes take place in cellular repair processes, genes, and hormones. When people fast, their blood sugars and insulin levels balance out. They also experience a drastic increase in their production of human growth hormone, which is responsible for repairing the body and supporting it in various healing processes.

Intermittent fasting is typically done for three reasons: to lose weight, to improve metabolic processes, or to protect against diseases. Some people will also do it simply because it is more convenient than cooking and sitting down to three or more meals per day.

Because of its ability to support your body in leveling out hormonal production and cellular repair, intermittent fasting is said to protect you against various diseases. Some of these include type 2 diabetes, heart disease, Alzheimer's disease, and even cancer. This alone can be reason enough for many to choose to eat this way.

What Should You Eat?

When it comes to intermittent fasting, the diet itself does not state what you should or should not eat. Instead, it is focused on when you should and should not eat. However, there are some things that you need to consider whenever it comes to consuming foods that are meant to support your health. This is especially true if you are choosing this diet with the sole purpose of supporting your health, which many do.

Depending on what your health goals are, you will want to pick foods accordingly. Typically, keeping plenty of organic vegetables and meat in your diet is a good idea.

Making sure that you pick nutritious, wholesome food choices that are rich with vitamins and minerals will ensure that you have plenty to keep you healthy.

If you are someone with specific dietary concerns or preferences, you can easily work that into your intermittent fasting diet. Due to the versatility of this diet, virtually any eating requirements and preferences can be accommodated for. Simply adjust your menu accordingly and make sure that you are eating enough during the non-fasting hours to keep your nutrition up and you will maintain great health with this diet.

Who Invented The Intermittent Fasting Diet?

The intermittent fasting diet has always been around in one way or another but was outlined as a specific dietary style and popularized back in 2012. The 5:2 adaptation of the intermittent fasting diet became popular in the UK after it was featured on a documentary that promoted the diet. It then snowballed into a widely practiced diet that has changed the lives of many different people.

Since the introduction of the 5:2 adaptation, many other adaptations such as the 16:8 and the alternating adaptations have been introduced. Each of these are intended to support individuals in getting the best benefits based on their unique needs and considerations.

What Do I Need To Consider?

As is true with anything when you are making changes to your health regimen, it is always a good idea to consult your doctor before trying the intermittent fasting diet. While fasting is natural for humans to participate in, extended or excessive fasting may not be healthy for all individuals. For example, those who are at risk of binge eating habits or eating disorders should avoid this diet as it may promote these behaviors in certain people.

Another time where intermittent fasting may not be ideal is if you already live with a disease such as a type 1 diabetes. These types of diseases often need to be managed and monitored with very strict dietary practices, so adjusting or changing your diet may not be ideal for you. This is especially true without the support of your physician.

In order to remain safe and to prevent experiencing any negative side effects, it is important that you consult with your physician first. This can support you in ensuring that intermittent fasting is safe for you, as well as assist you in learning more about specific nutritional considerations that you need to consider for yourself.

Other individuals, such as pregnant women and those who are breastfeeding should also be cautious when practicing diets such as intermittent fasting. Again, pregnancy and breastfeeding are two times in a woman's life where specific nutritional requirements generally need to be considered to maintain your health. Consulting with your doctor can help you decide what is right and safe for you and your baby.

Chapter 2 Why Intermittent Fasting is Superior

Intermittent fasting is superior to virtually every other diet in many different ways. The nature of this diet is significantly different from the nature of other diets that people typically choose. Because of how this diet is structured, with a greater emphasis on when food is consumed versus what food is consumed, it provides more benefits than most conventional diets do.

It is More Convenient

The intermittent fasting diet is widely touted for its many health benefits, but it has some other benefits, too. For example, the intermittent fasting diet is convenient. When you eat this way, you do not have to spend quite as much time cooking, eating, and cleaning. Instead of eating several meals per day, most intermittent fasters only eat one or two big meals and then a few snacks.

Less time preparing and planning for meal times means that you can spend more time doing other things. For example, if you are someone who likes to sleep in but has to be at the office early, you can skip over breakfast and catch some extra sleep each morning. This won't have any negative benefits on your health because you are simply eating in accordance with your diet. Furthermore, it may actually improve your mood because you go the extra rest that you needed before you left!

You Can Eat What You Want

One of the reasons why the intermittent fasting diet is so great is that you can still eat virtually anything you want on this diet. While this is not a reason to get silly with the desserts and go overboard on junk foods, you also do not have to worry about restricting yourself to just one cookie, or a 1/8" piece of cake at dessert. Instead, you can enjoy the full piece or a couple of cookies and have no worries about any repercussions that you may face.

This also means that all of your favorite recipes that you have fallen in love with over the years are still useable and you do not have to completely overhaul your entire recipe book. Rather than having to learn and attempt to like all new recipes, you can continue loving the ones you always have. Then, you can add newer ones when you want to, not because you have to.

The fact that you can continue eating how you want when you eat according to the intermittent fasting diet makes this diet more sustainable than others. Other diets often require you to cut out certain things or reduce the types of food that you eat. As a result, many individuals find themselves craving these things since they have typically eaten them for a long time. Attempting to stay true to their diet, they will often deny themselves the indulgence until they can no longer stand it and they cave. Then, they typically cave to the point that they talk themselves into staying off of their diet for a while. This can lead to losing the results they gained, as well as feeling badly about themselves.

Instead of attempting to stick yourself to a diet that does not truly give you the foods you want to be eating, intermittent fasting allows you to eat as you normally would. You simply include fasting windows so that you can gain the health benefits without enduring drastic changes to your favorite menus.

Eating Out is Still a Breeze

One thing that many other diets do not accommodate for is eating out. Attempting to eat out when you are on a diet can be challenging. Choosing restaurants that serve foods that accommodate your needs or attempting to educate your friends and family on what you can and cannot have can be frustrating. It can cause people to avoid going out because they do not want to be a hassle to their loved ones or struggle to find something to eat at a restaurant.

When you are on the intermittent fasting diet, eating out is still an easy task. Rather than having to research restaurants to find ones that you can eat at or attempt to get loved ones to change their menus for you, you can simply go enjoy yourself. As long as you are not going out to eat during a fasting window, there are no restrictions that you need to worry about. This makes dining out much easier.

Prevents You from Eating Dangerous Diets

Many people look to dieting as a way to improve their health and reach their health goals. It is to be expected, too. What we eat has a major impact on our overall health. It is no secret that eating properly can support you in having improved health and a greater quality of life. However, many people choose to diet in a way that can actually have a negative impact on them.

It is not uncommon for people to follow fad diets as a way to attempt to improve their health using all of the "latest research." Many of these diets are not actually sustainable, as they require strict practices that prevent people from feeling satisfied and nourished after their meals. As a result, people find themselves struggling to maintain the diet. Furthermore, they may find themselves feeling more irritable and frustrated with themselves rather than empowered and proud of themselves. This can lead to many psychological issues, too.

Eating the intermittent fasting diet is more about a lifestyle change than a diet. Because you still have a great deal of flexibility in what you can eat, you do not have to worry about trying to consume things according to a strict menu. As a result, you can enjoy eating everything that makes you feel satisfied. You simply wait until your "eating window" before starting. This makes the diet much more sustainable and prevents dangerous yo-yo dieting or following fad diets that could result in malnourishment and frustration.

Chapter 3 How Intermittent Fasting Benefits Your Health

Right now, we have a global epidemic of obesity and diabetes plaguing our society physically, emotionally and financially. In fact, approximately 2.8 million people globally die every year to obesity-related illnesses according to the WHO. Not only does this mean an early grave, but it can also mean a lifelong struggle and disability. Issues like diabetes, ischemic heart disease, certain cancers, and an array of health problems can all be attributed to Obesity. Some unfortunate individuals are born with predispositions to these diseases; however, a vast majority can be attributed to lifelong eating habits. Eating highly processed foods full of saturated fat and LDL Cholesterol throughout the entire day maintaining your body's fed state is a key contributor to developing obesity. If you eat like this, not only are you forming a mitochondrial addiction as your insulin levels constantly spike throughout the day, but you are accompanying that with artery clogging, brain damaging and cancer-causing substances.

So how does Intermittent fasting help with all of this? Firstly, we will cover the physical health benefits then move on to the beneficial mental results you can achieve from it. These are things such as undergoing healthy weight loss. Let us start with the metabolic disease Diabetes. Someone has Diabetes when their body does not produce enough or any insulin and/or when their body's cells do not know how to react to insulin. This inadequacy of insulin can leave individuals with dangerously high glucose levels in their blood. Intermittent fasting lets you better control insulin levels actually. The World Journal of Diabetes found that intermittent fasting on a regular basis helped reduce post-meal glucose spikes.

Healthy Weight Loss

One of the most commonly known benefits from intermittent fasting is the healthy weight loss. With this weight loss also comes improvements to your cardiovascular health and your gut health. The weight loss will almost be immediate once you start practicing a periodic fasting regimen due to the inevitable lower caloric intake. We will discuss more about caloric intake later on. In a systematic review of 40 unique intermittent fasting studies, the average weight loss recorded was 7-11 pounds over 10 weeks. Take note that the participants ranged in size from lean to obese.

Leaner individuals will typically experience a less drastic weight loss compared to their larger counterparts. Losing excess weight comes with more benefits for your cardiovascular system. Things like hypertension, which are three times more prevalent in obese individuals, and congestive heart failure have been found to have a direct correlation with being overweight and obese.

According to the American Heart Association, for patients experiencing these problems, "reductions in weight dramatically improve ventricular function and oxygenation." However, it is not just the heart; your gut will benefit too. Our gut is actually much more complex than you may assume. In every human gut, there live thousands of species like bacteria, viruses, fungi, and amoebae. These microbes can actually alter how we metabolize our foods, and even alter how they tell our body when it should feel hungry. These complex communities of microbes change over time and can be directly affected by the environment they are subject to. In 2017, a study in cell metabolism found that there was an increase in the fermentation products acetate and lactate that help fat cells produce more mitochondria. Increased mitochondria of these cells mean stored fat is being used as energy more than before. An almost guaranteed benefit you can get from intermittent fasting is weight loss and thus significantly reducing your risk to any of this issue and ailments.

Healthy Skin

Then there is the outside of your body, the part that everybody sees every day, your skin. Your skin can be a clear indicator of how your body is in that moment and it can reflect how it has been treated. Constantly being in a fed state can put a lot of stress on your body as it is always focused on digesting your last meal. Stress can represent itself in so many ways including blotchy skin, redness, inflammation, and acne. Coupled with a diet high in saturated fat and processed oils, you would be lucky not to show any signs. Intermittent fasting not only allows your body to completely digest food then focus on functioning optimally but also typically increases the amount of water you will drink. Women need more water as is due to the estrogen and progesterone that lowers blood plasma volumes, and in turn, can bring on quicker fatigue or dehydration. While intermittent fasting, you will be drinking significantly more water throughout the week which comes with its own plethora of benefits for the skin and rest of your body.

When your body is focusing on digesting in a fed state, it is also in a parasympathetic state through your automatic nervous system (ANS). Your ANS has two states as well, sympathetic and parasympathetic. The sympathetic nervous system is active when you are in "fight or flight" mode, basically, anytime you are actively using your skeletal muscles. The parasympathetic state is when you are in a "rest and digest" mode and your body's energy is going towards the internal functioning of digestive organs. Staying a Fed and Parasympathetic state continuously can lead to negative effects on your mood, motivation, brain health, and sleep. Studies done by the University of Virginia concluded that consistent IF [might] improve cognitive functions and brain structures.

Better Sleep

Intermittent fasting can also improve your sleeping patterns. However, have you ever actually tried sleeping on an empty stomach? It is hard, isn't it? That is because most of us are so used to being in that fed state, basically having a full stomach, and our systems are literally depending on more energy from food entering the body. However, after the initial adjustment period, fasting has shown to be able to improve sleep quality in a variety of studies. One group of researchers and experts in particular in the Dept. of Internal Medicine at Kliniken Essen Mitte in Germany conducted an open pilot study that was able to come to this conclusion disturbances in sleeping patterns are lowered hence the night time rests are peaceful and uninterrupted. The one-week long fasting aided in this and in effect, the energy levels and strength of these individuals belonging to normal BMI levels are better more than ever in their day-to-day activities. What is particularly useful about this study is that 92% of the test subjects were women. They measured sleep patterns of these women using polysomnography.

Polysomnography is a widely used method of diagnosing sleep disorders and monitoring sleep patterns. It is done by measuring the brain waves, oxygen levels, eye, and facial twitching, the heartbeat, breathing patterns, and any muscle movements of the subject as they sleep. Once you get yourself over the adjustment period, you can expect to see improvements in your morning mood and energy. It is important to note their findings on obese subjects too. It's one theory that the practice of periodic or intermittent fasting triggered both weight loss, reduced stress on the body from constantly combating glucose spikes and allowed the individuals parasympathetic nervous system to diet all functions to obtaining adequate rest for the body, as opposed to digesting food and adjust blood sugar levels during their sleep.

Intermittent fasting comes with this array of benefits and reduces risk to so many preventable diseases, but it is not to be taken lightly. If done wrong you can endanger yourself, so you have to take the right precautions when deciding to live this way. You should consider all personal circumstances too. Nevertheless, if you think you're ready, it is time to pick a method and make it yours! For a quick reference of some the benefits intermittent fasting can bring you, check out the graphic on the next page.

Which Women Should Avoid or Be Extra Cautious About Intermittent Fasting?

Depending on what stage of life you are in and your special circumstances, any form of intermittent fasting might not be for you. Any form of fasting is not recommended if you are breastfeeding or pregnant. When you are pregnant, the food you will be consuming is for two individuals and fasting can cause a high risk for potential harm to the fetus. Healthy fetal development depends on a wide range of hormones and their processes can heavily depend on the functioning of the parts of your brain important for hormones. These hormonal glands are going to be affected directly during a fast due to the inevitably lower insulin levels you will have. Intermittent fasting can affect every woman differently, but the adverse short-term effects are relatively benign. When you are pregnant, those short-term adverse effects can be life-threatening for the fetus and potentially permanently damaging.

Diseases like metabolic syndrome, when your body's metabolism is messed up in one way or another, are rooted in how insulin acts in your body and insulin is the most important hormone affected by any fasting regimen.

Chapter 4 Impact of Intermittent Fasting on Your Body

Intermittent fasting has several positive effects on the body. It helps in bringing your physiological functions in sync. You start feeling more alert, fit, and healthy. The feelings of lethargy and fatigue go away. Your body starts responding to exercise very well. You lose weight fast and feel good. It also has an anti-aging effect and you feel younger inside out. These things happen when you start following a set intermittent fasting protocol and make some positive changes in your food and eating habits. Our body has a great ability to resolve most of the health issues if it gets the right environment and intermittent fasting provides your body with the same.

The following are some of the most important effects of intermittent fasting.

Promotes Fat Burning

Fat accumulation is a simple process for your body. Whatever you eat gets converted into glucose that is released into your bloodstream. Your body can use this glucose directly as energy. So, whenever you eat anything, the food gets processed and the energy in the form of glucose mixes with your blood and raises your blood sugar levels. The pancreas in the body senses the increase in blood sugar level and pumps out insulin hormone to stabilize the blood sugar levels. Insulin is a chemical messenger that communicates with the cells and helps them in absorbing the glucose. It is also the main fat storage hormone of your body. It binds with the cells and allows them to absorb the required energy. The surplus energy is then stored in the muscles and liver in form of glycogen. The glycogen stores are individual power stores of the muscles where they are stored. Muscles can use these stores whenever needed however the glycogen stores of one muscle cannot be used for others. The liver can use its glycogen stores for supplying energy to other organs. However, there is a limit to the amount of energy that can be stored even in form of glycogen. The insulin in your body then starts storing the surplus energy in form of fat.

As soon as insulin level in your bloodstream rises your body gets a message that it needs to store energy. It gets in the energy hoarding mode and it will not be inclined to burn fat. It is a simple way of prioritizing. If there is any energy need, it will be fulfilled from the surplus energy present at disposal and in no case, the stored energy will be used. This makes losing weight while having continuously high levels of insulin in your bloodstream very difficult. The whole process is working against your weight loss goals. You will have to work extra hard and will have to spend more energy than you have consumed. It may also lead to fatigue and exhaustion.

Now let's suppose you had your last meal at least 14 hours ago at 6 O' Clock in the evening. At 8 O' Clock in the morning, the insulin levels in your blood would be very low. Your body would already be looking for energy. It needs a steady supply of energy to run various functions. As soon as energy supply gets thin and the demand escalates, your body starts looking for alternate energy sources. Glycogen is an easy source of energy, but one muscle cannot donate its glycogen to another, hence it isn't readily available for use. In such a situation, the body starts producing fat burning hormones like the growth hormone. This hormone enables the metabolization of the fat stores and your body would automatically start burning the fat even if you do no workout.

So, by not eating the food for a few hours, you will be actually helping your body in metabolizing the fat. All your weight loss efforts will be fully supported by your body as it would also want to use that fat for energy and wouldn't be in a fat storage mode as usually happens while you do exercise in your normal routine. Through intermittent fasting, you can promote fat burning process in your body. Even a small effort will mean more as no counterproductive process will be going in your body that leads to fat storage.

Boosts Growth Hormone Production

The growth hormone is one of the most amazing hormones in the body. Our body produces this hormone in large quantities in our formative years. It helps in tissue and bone growth. The strength in the bones comes with the help of this hormone. It plays a vital role in protein synthesis and muscle building. It means that if the levels of growth hormone are high in your blood, you would be able to build muscles comparatively faster.

It also enables fat breakdown for releasing energy. Here, it is important to understand that there are certain important pre-requisites for the production of growth hormone in your body. The first is that insulin levels in your bloodstream must be very low. The production of growth hormone is high when you are feeling hungry. When you feel hunger, your gut releases the 'ghrelin' hormone which is the hunger hormone. It increases the production of growth hormone so that energy deficit can be compensated by metabolizing the fat stores. So, if fat reduction is your goal, you must ensure that your body naturally keeps producing growth hormone in good quantity. The production of growth hormone is also the highest when you are asleep. To sum up, if you ate early in the evening and slept, during the wee hours, your body will be producing growth hormones in large quantities.

Growth hormone has some very unique functions. It helps in the growth of all internal organs in your body including your brain. It also strengthens your immune system and beefs up your protection mechanism. You also get better healing powers. Even your sex life would improve as growth hormone has a strong effect on your mood and sexual performance. Men suffering from erectile dysfunction notice considerable improvement and women facing the loss of libido also start enjoying their sex life better.

Growth hormone also improves your cardiovascular function as it helps in removing bad cholesterol and triglycerides. Your sleep patterns improve when your growth hormone level is high. Even your mood also improves a lot with its growth.

The production of this hormone is not always the same in our body. During childhood, the production of this hormone is high, it peaks out when you hit puberty as your body goes through a lot of natural changes. In teenage, the production of growth hormone remains high as you are still growing but your body reduces the production of growth hormone once you cross teenage.

Your body still needs immunity, tissue and muscle building, and other such things and that's why the production of growth hormone is there in spurts when the conditions are right. If you can naturally create the conditions which help in the production of growth hormone, fighting obesity and other diseases will become very easy. You will also be able to build muscles and get better results from your exercise routines.

This is where intermittent fasting comes into play. Intermittent fasting helps your body in creating the natural energy deficit and keeps you in the fasted state for longer periods. When you fast for longer than 8-12 hours your insulin levels go down. Your body also starts releasing the ghrelin hormone which is a message to your brain to eat. It is generally advised to eat a few hours before your bedtime so that you are still asleep when this whole process is going inside your body. In this state, you would also not be able to feel the intensity of hunger and hence there will not be any craving for food. Your body will be able to produce the growth hormone in large quantities.

Well researched studies have shown that women practicing intermittent fasting can experience a 1300% growth in the production of growth hormone in their body. This is not all, the production of growth hormone in men practicing intermittent fasting can get even higher up to 2000%. This can be the single most important thing that should be enough motivation for intermittent fasting. It can help you in leading a healthier and better life. You will not only be able to fight obesity with greater ease but you will also be able to achieve holistic overall health.

The importance of growth hormone in development and fat loss has been understood by the whole world it is among the leading causes of the use of synthetic growth hormone injection. However, not only the use of synthetic growth hormone prohibited by law, but it is also very dangerous. The structure of synthetic growth hormone is very different to the one produced by our body and hence it causes more harm than good.

Intermittent fasting is the easiest and the safest way to lose excess fat, and become healthy. You can get all the benefits of growth hormone by simply following an intermittent fasting routine. If you do high-intensity exercises in the morning in the fasted state, your fat loss abilities, as well as muscle building power, would increase tremendously. During exercise, you lose a lot of muscle but the presence of growth hormone ensures that the recovery is fast and better.

If you are concerned whether you will be able to do an intense workout or not on an empty, you do not need to worry at all. High-intensity exercises target specific muscles and the muscles have their own glycogen stores for energy. You would feel no dearth of energy even in the fasted state. Besides that, when your body starts burning the fat fuel, it releases a lot of energy. It is more efficient and cleaner fuel for your body that emits the least amount of toxic waste. Therefore, apart from the initial few days while you are getting used to the routine, you will never feel energy drained or exhausted due to the fasts.

If you are following an unhealthy lifestyle which involves erratic eating patterns your growth hormone production will be very low. Common symptoms of growth hormone deficiency are:

- *Depression*
- *Sexual dysfunction*
- *Hair loss*
- *Decreases muscle strength and mass*
- *Dry skin*
- *Temperature sensitivities*
- *Lack of concentration*
- *Memory loss*
- *Increased weight and protruding belly*
- *Insulin resistance*
- *Fatigue*
- *High triglycerides*
- *Low LDL (Bad Cholesterol)*
- *High risk of heart diseases*

The production of growth hormone goes down as you advance in age and that is a natural process. However, when coupled with other problems like insulin resistance, high stress, and liver malfunction, the problems become big. Intermittent fasting is an easy and natural way to increase the production of growth hormone in your body. You will feel much better, healthier, stronger, and will also be able to bring your waistline down.

Prevents Insulin Resistance

The beauty of nature is in balance and even the human body follows the same rule. Whenever there is an imbalance in any process, it has a very adverse impact on our health. The same is the case with insulin hormone. Insulin is a very important hormone. It is crucial for processing blood sugar in your body. The pancreas starts releasing insulin as soon as you consume food. The levels of insulin are at peak in your blood immediately after any meal and they are the lowest 8-12 hours after your last meal. When you consume meals at regular intervals of 3-4 hours in a day, the pancreas never stops releasing insulin. It is forced to continuously release insulin in short spurts.

The perineal presence of insulin in your blood triggers another big problem and that's insulin resistance. Insulin resistance is a stage when your cells stop binding readily with insulin. When insulin levels in your blood remain consistently high, your body starts showing indifference towards it. As a result, your pancreas needs to release more insulin to process the same amount of blood sugar. It starts a vicious cycle. Your body is not able to burn fat as high insulin levels in your blood support fat storage in place of fat burning. Your body reacts slow to insulin and hence your body needs to produce more insulin. This leads to pre-diabetes.

Around 100 million people in the US are currently affected with prediabetes. It is the beginning stage of most of the health issues and will later on become Type-II diabetes. It is a preventable problem and yet so many people get affected by it every year.

Intermittent fasting can help you in preventing pre-diabetes to a great extent. It allows your body to remain in the fasted state for at least 14 hours a day. After your last meal, the insulin concentration in your blood becomes very low in 8-12 hours. This helps in developing insulin sensitivity in the body. The cells become more responsive to insulin. Your pancreas does not need to continuously pump insulin into your blood and hence the pressure on the pancreas also goes down. This starts a very positive chain of events that will prevent your body from excessive stress and dangers of insulin resistance. You can bring this change by simply altering your eating and fasting pattern.

Reduces the Risk of Heart Diseases

Heart diseases are among the biggest reasons for preventable deaths in the US. The prevalence of heart diseases has increased a lot in the past few decades and the main reason for it is a poor lifestyle. There is a lot of stress, poor eating habits and unhealthy choice of food items that increase the risk of heart diseases many times.

The main reason for most of the heart problems is an imbalance in the levels of HDL (Good Cholesterol), LDL (Bad Cholesterol) and Triglycerides. It is a building block of many important things. However, the increase in the ratio of LDL and triglycerides can spell a problem for you. LDL is a low-density lipoprotein that gets deposited in your arteries and it can choke it. High deposit of LDL also leads to high blood pressure levels. It hardens your arteries and narrows them. It can also lead to the formation of blood clots that would obstruct the flow of blood.

People mostly believe that if they do not eat food items that are high on cholesterol, they would remain safe. However, it isn't the case. Dietary cholesterol has a minimal role to play in the process and most of the cholesterol comes from the fat in your body. Your fat cells keep releasing the cholesterol for various functions. The greater the amount of fat in the body, the higher your cholesterol levels would be. This would also increase the risk of heart diseases for you.

The real problem lies in the way our body is treating components like LDL, VLDL, and triglycerides. While you are on a regular diet, your body is using sugar as the main fuel source. The glucose is easy to burn and therefore, your body wouldn't use fat as fuel. However, when you make some dietary changes and follow intermittent fasting you force your body to burn the fat fuel. When you eat anything it gets converted into energy. Some of it is used while most of it is stored in some form or the other. Your body converts the energy into triglycerides that are a form of lipid and then stores them in fat cells.

This increases the level of triglycerides in your blood. Your body is regularly synthesizing the free-fatty acids called triglycerides. Your liver, on the other hand, has to continuously produce VLDL to transport triglycerides and cholesterol to various parts.

When you start following an intermittent fasting protocol, you force your body to burn fat. This means that your body would start using the triglycerides in place of making them. They form a major part of the problem. When your triglyceride levels go down, your VLDL levels would also go down as your liver would have to produce less VLDL to transport triglycerides. This would also lower your LDL levels.

In this whole process, the levels of HDL, the good cholesterol would remain the same in your blood. This cholesterol has the ability to clean the plaque deposits in your arteries and keep your heart healthy. High HDL and low LDL means your heart health would remain good.

You can bring this positive change in your life by simply adopting a healthy lifestyle change, a good and nutritious diet, and an intermittent fasting protocol.

Increases Metabolic Rate

Metabolic rate is a common term people hear when talking about weight loss. In simple terms, metabolism is the speed at which your body is utilizing the nutrition. It means if your metabolism is high, your body will be consuming more calories and producing more energy. You will feel fit and agile. If your metabolism is slow, your body will not be able to process the energy fast. Your per day calorie consumption would get low. You will feel lethargic, tired, uninterested, and unmotivated. Metabolism is the key to weight management and hence having a high metabolism is very important.

Starvation diets or the diets which impose strict calorie restrictions actually lower your metabolic rate. Your body stops getting the required amount of nutrition and therefore it slows the energy consumption speed. You would start feeling lethargic, tired and may experience fatigue but the weight loss would be minimal.

The metabolic rate in our body is the number of calories it burns in a unit of time. Either you are working, standing, playing, eating, or sleeping, your body never stops working. It continuously needs the energy to run various organs. Out of the total energy that is required, your liver alone uses 27% of the energy, the brain takes another 19% of the total energy. Even processing the food that you eat requires burning some calories and the percentage is around 10% of your daily spend.

If your metabolic rate is high, you will be able to burn a greater number of calories in the same amount of time in a day and hence lose weight. Sitting idle and stressing out can lower your metabolism rate. Your metabolism can also go down due to some other factors too like chronic diseases, medication, hormonal imbalance, etc.

The metabolic rate of healthy individuals is higher than the overweight ones. The reason is simple, muscles utilize more energy than the fat cells. So, the greater the amount of fat in the body the lower the metabolic rate would be. It would also make losing weight difficult as the energy demands of your body go down. You can change this by slowly increasing the energy demands of your body. Junk food that is full of empty calories will always slow down your metabolism. It leads to greater fat deposit. If you want to increase your metabolism, you must focus on clean eating. The more nutritious food you eat, the better your metabolism would be.

Exercise is also a great way to increase your metabolic rate. It creates a huge energy demand and your body starts using surplus energy. Stable sleep patterns are also very helpful in improving the metabolic rate.

Intermittent fasting is another great way to boost your metabolic rate. Studies have shown that intermittent fasting can boost metabolic rate by 10%. This is a huge jump if you want to lose weight and reduce your waistline.

Intermittent fasting creates an energy deficit while ensuring that you get your daily requirement of macronutrients, vitamins, and minerals. It also helps in the production of some crucial hormones that help in increasing the metabolic rate.

Frequent eating puts a lot of pressure on your body to process that energy. It is one of the reasons that people start feeling drowsy after having a heavy meal. Your body needs time to transport that energy to various parts of the body. Surplus energy makes the process very inefficient and fat deposits increase.

Intermittent fasting creates the energy gap and your body starts processing the energy more efficiently. Your metabolic rate increases and it also helps you in losing weight.

Chapter 5 Fasting for Weight Loss

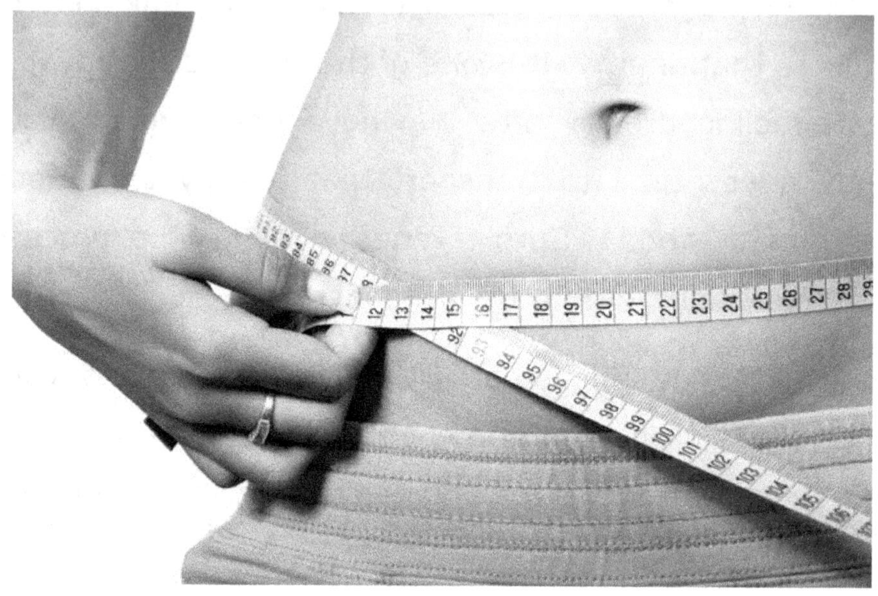

There are so many different reasons why we all gain weight. Some people think everyone that is obese sits around eating junk all day. Sure, maybe some do this, but in general, there is usually an underlying health reason that someone might have struggles when trying to lose weight and reduce their overall weight gain.

As we mentioned earlier, when you are overweight, it will be even harder for you to try and reduce that weight and easier for your body to start to pack on even more pounds. One of the reasons that you might have trouble losing weight is because of your body's natural tendency to retain water.

Cause of Weight Gain

If you are eating foods that are high in salt, then this can cause your body to hold onto a lot of weight through excess water. This will usually show itself in visual places, such as your chin/chest, your feet, or your hands. When you first start on a healthy diet, you might drop 20 pounds in as quick as a month.

This is because your body is letting go of that water. Then, as weight loss progresses, it becomes a lot slower, because you're not holding onto that water. This can be very discouraging for some. They might start a drastic diet, losing five pounds in just a week. Then, however, they might gain back three pounds the next week, and think that the diet doesn't work, quitting, and moving on. Always remember water retention in the struggle for weight loss.

Our bodies can sometimes resist our attempt at weight loss as well. If you are participating in extreme diets like only drinking lemon water for a week, but then go back to eating unhealthily next week, you're confusing your body. It will resist that diet in the first place in order to better deal with the fluctuations you're seeing. This is why you might feel like you gain weight quickly, or why if you lose weight, it doesn't always stay off.

Another cause of weight gain can be not eating right, along with exercising. You might be an active person, or know an active person, who frequently works out or participate in sports. Despite their dedication, they're still overweight. The biggest reason for this is unhealthy eating. Some people can get away with eating unhealthily and exercising and still having a low body weight and fit physique. However, for the most part, it's crucial that we also focus on healthier diets in addition to whichever workout we choose to add.

Alternatively, some people think they don't have to exercise at all, and the weight will just come off. In the beginning, this is true. If you don't work out and don't eat healthily, but then start to eat healthy food, you will lose some weight. You will eventually plateau, however, especially after your stomach and metabolism adjust. Not everyone has to dedicate an hour a day at the gym. However, light and frequent cardio, such as a walk every other day or 20 minutes on the treadmill a day are still very important if you want to lose weight continually.

There are many sneaky foods that will get into our diets and cause us to hang onto unwanted weight as well. The biggest hidden food is sugar. This will often be found in highly processed foods. Some things might market themselves as organic, making you think "healthy." They might also show pictures of fruits and veggies, stating things like "contains two whole apples, one berry, one banana, etc." What they won't put on the front, however, is that they also contain %30 of your daily recommended sugar!

Things like yogurt, deli meats, frozen veggies, and other processed foods that are seemingly harmless might very well contain high levels of sodium, which will cause water retention, and high levels of sugar, which can imbalance your hormones and cause a higher amount of fat to be stored throughout your body.

Dehydration is another culprit of obesity. Water needs to be consumed in certain amounts depending on your body weight, regardless if you drink other beverages. Some people might think that they had some coffee, juice, tea, or even a soda, and think this counts towards their hydration level. However, some of these will contain things that can even dehydrate you further, so it's crucial that you never deprive yourself an excessive amount of water.

One of the biggest reasons that we might struggle with obesity and the overall ability to lose weight is because of the mentality around dieting. To lose weight doesn't mean to give up food for a month, and then the pounds come off and stay off. There's no pill, shake, or surgery that will help you stay in shape. These things will remove fat, but they won't keep them off and can end up causing you to gain more weight later on because of the intense fluctuation in debt we're giving our bodies. If you really want to lose weight and fight obesity, then we need to work with our body's natural fat-burning properties.

A Healthy and Balanced Diet

Fasting is a great way to lose weight. However, if you are eating unhealthy during the periods that you do eat, then fasting isn't going to end up doing you any good. Your body will eventually balance out.

You should be eating a balanced diet even if you read this book through and then decide fasting isn't for you. The combination of both, along with exercise, is going to be your secret to melting your body fat, however. Throughout this chapter, we are going to take a look at some of the best ways that you can burn your body fat through a healthy and balanced diet.

The biggest mistake dieters will make is by purchasing and focusing only on "diet," "organic," "natural," and other types of foods that are only labeled for being healthy. Don't be misguided by some fancy wording, especially blank statements like "part of a complete meal." Any meal could be complete! "Part of a healthy meal," is something that is actually saying something of value.

Start by cutting out as many processed foods as possible. We'll all have those pizza cravings after a night out at the bar or want to indulge in a sugary coffee with our breakfasts. However, you should be putting an emphasis on having these things as treats. If you have them every once in a while, your body will be able to process them easier, meaning it's not like you'll gain two pounds from having one slice of cake. However, if you have a slice of cake every day, you will start to gain weight again. Don't think you have to cut them out of your life altogether – this is the kind of all or nothing thinking that can send us into a panic and want to binge.

Of course, you might struggle with your control over food and find it difficult to have "just a few" of certain kinds of sweets. Still, make it a priority to reduce the number of junk food items you add in regularly.

Choose whole wheat over white carbs, such as whole-wheat bread versus white bread, whole-grain pasta over white pasta, and so on. Pick lean meat like chicken and fish over heavier red meat like bacon and steak.

Pick fresh fruits and veggies over canned, and make sure if you do buy frozen that there are no additives. Always check your labels and make sure the sugar, salt, and fat content are lower than other vitamin and mineral counts that might be labeled.

Don't think you can't snack either. Smaller meals combined with healthier snacks throughout the day is always a better choice than just three huge meals.

Regulating Your Metabolism

The reason that some people will include cheat days in their diet is first to alleviate some of the pressures of dieting and give into their biggest cravings. It's also helpful in keeping your metabolism on its toes. Combined with fasting, this will help keep your metabolism active and regulated rather than sticking to one diet, and one kind of food, all the time.

Your metabolism is based on weight, age, and sex. The younger you are, the bigger you are, and the more muscles you have, the faster you burn food. Men typically have more muscles than women (think hips/breasts/and other fatty areas on women), which is why it might be easier for a husband to lose weight after giving up soda, while his wife struggles to lose a pound even though she eats nothing but salad. The combination of a balanced diet with fasting will help to keep your metabolism regulated.

How to Use Fasting for Weight Loss

All of this means that adding fasting to whatever else you are doing will help you to lose weight. The more of these healthy habits you can add into your life, such as focusing on balanced meals and exercise, the better results you will see.

Fasting can burn fat, detoxify your body, and help build self-control. All of this can lead to a healthier lifestyle you've been looking for.

Chapter 6 Fasting and female hormones

Intermittent fasting has shown to affect females' hormones, and there are some things women need to consider before they start fasting. Some studies are showing how intermittent fasting can negatively impact the female's reproductive system, and the reason why these shifts occur is that women are sensitive to lower calorie intake.

Hypothalamus can disrupt the production of gonadotropin-releasing hormone (GnRH), which is responsible for releasing the two reproductive hormones, luteinizing hormone (LH) and follicle stimulating hormone (FSH). Once these hormones have been affected negatively from an extended period by restricting calories, you will be running a risk of irregular periods, infertility, poor bone health, and other health risks. Even though autophagy has shown to do the opposite, it puts women in a complicated situation when it comes to fasting. For that reason, we don't recommend women fast for more than 24 hours as it can affect women hormone in a very drastic manner.

Instead, women should use a modified approach that we talked about in this book. To make sure women don't notice any hormone imbalance, fast alternate days instead of back to back, keeping you in a safe place. If you want to fast aggressively for weight loss, then our recommendation is not to prolong it for more than 4-6 weeks. But then again, make sure you consult a professional before you may start fasting as everybody is different. On the plus side, there are many benefits women will notice if they begin fasting the right way. As we know, heart disease is killing people every day, in one study done on obese women showed that intermittent fasting lowered LDL cholesterol or which is the leading cause of heart problems in North America.

Also, intermittent fasting has shown to make you more insulin sensitive. In one study of 100 obese women showed that six months of intermittent fasting reduced insulin levels by 29% and insulin resistance by 19 %, although blood sugar remained the same. Having higher sensitively to insulin has shown to lower the risk of type 2 diabetes, but intermittent fasting may not be beneficial for women as it is for men in regards to blood sugar. In mice, it has been shown to increase the longevity by 33% although long term studies on humans are yet to be determined.

Finally, intermittent fasting can reduce inflammation levels. Even though more studies need to be executed for women and intermittent fasting, it is pretty clear that there are hosts of benefits if done right. As long as you are taking intermittent fasting the right way, and you are not abusing it, your hormones should be in check. Remember, if you are pregnant, this might affect you very differently. Moreover, we do not recommend women fast when they are pregnant or trying to conceive, but as long as you know the repercussions of fasting too long.

Why intermittent fasting effects women's hormone more than men's?

If you have been doing research online, then you might have read claims such as "intermittent fasting is not for women" or "if women intermittent fast, their hormones will be out of whack." Which isn't the case, as we will discuss how intermittent fasting truly affects women's hormone as when compared to men.

To briefly talk about men, they were created to "hunt and gather" so to speak. Unlike women, they do not have to carry a baby, which is one of the reasons why intermittent fasting does not affect men as drastically as women.

The good news is, it will not affect your thyroid as some "experts" will claim, women recognize hunger at a higher degree than men. We recently talked about the Hypothalamus gonadotropin-releasing hormone (GnRH), luteinizing hormone (LH) and follicle stimulating hormone (FSH), which is responsible for making testosterone and sperm in men and triggering estrogen and ovulation in women.

Women tend to trigger these hormones differently when compared to men, and the main problem occurs because of kisspeptin. For readers that don't know what kisspeptin is, it is a protein like molecules that neurons use to communicate with each other. Women tend to produce more kisspeptin when compared to men, which is a precursor to (GnRH).

As you know (GnRH) is going to dictate how women produce estrogen and how men are going to produce testosterone; another thing is that kisspeptin is very sensitive to the hunger hormone. The reason behind is kisspeptin, which causes women to produce less kisspeptin and leads to lower progesterone. In one study done on rats, showed that when female rats fast for one day which is more like a week for women, it caused them to lose 19% of their body weight but their ovaries shrunk significantly.

Also, they noticed that female rats luteinizing hormone plummeted, and their estrogen levels went thru the roof. To briefly touch upon thyroid, t3 levels were deceased. But, t3 levels are always decreasing between meals. The t4 which is responsible for producing thyroid remained the same, which means the thyroid isn't being affected drastically. It is always suggested that you get regular blood work done to ensure your thyroid is fine, but one of them to tell if it isn't is by seeing how could you get.

If you feel cold all the time, then the chances are your thyroid is lower. If you notice that you are getting starving throughout the day, and it becomes tough to fast, then break the fast and try it again later. As women, you need to listen to your more than men, as women tend to be more sensitive to hormones when intermittent fasting.

Eating enough calories

Since you now know the science behind intermittent fasting and how it can affect women's hormone, let us talk about eating enough calories, especially for women. Believe it or not, this is an important topic to discuss.

Especially for women who are much more sensitive to hunger hormones or hormones in general when compared to men. Even though you might be fasting for weight loss, it is critical that you enough calories support your bodily function as a woman. Ideally speaking women who are trying to lose weight should not eat bellow 200 calories of their maintenance, calculating your maintenance calories the formula is (bodyweight x 12).

Meaning, if your maintenance calories are 2,000 and you are looking to lose weight, then you should not cut it down less than 1,800. If you are someone looking to lose weight with intermittent fasting, we recommend having a macronutrient break down of 20% carbs 50% protein and 30% fats; this shows the percentage of calories coming from specific macronutrients.

We are keeping the carbs low to prevent insulin spikes in check if you are looking to lose weight, we want to keep the insulin as flatlined as possible. However, if you are someone looking to maintain weight and reap the health benefits of intermittent fasting, then we recommend having a macronutrient breakdown of 30% carbs 40% protein 30% fats since we have covered the calorie intake, lets briefly talk about the types of food you should be eating. What you eat to break your fast is just as essential as the number of calories you should be consuming. One thing you need to understand is not to go overboard on the fasting.

As you know, carbs tend to spike your insulin, and when you're fasting, your insulin levels are low, meaning whatever you eat, your body will be sensitive to it. Having spikes of insulin slows down fat loss. Therefore, lower insulin equals more fat burning. If you break your fast with higher amounts of carbs, you will be shutting down the fat burning process. Instead, what we recommend is eating two meals when you break in your eating window. The first one should be lower in carbs and higher in fats and protein; this will ensure you don't turn off your fat burning and get the most out of your fast. The second meal could be higher carbs, and this will help you get ready for the next day if you are fasting.

Another to remember is that your gut will be susceptible to high acidic foods such and drinks, so make sure you stick to foods which are less acidic when you break your fast. Greek yogurt, chicken with some veggies or even soup works great to break your fast. Now whether your goal is to lose weight or live a healthier life, it is essential that you follow the right calorie intake and macronutrients intake. These tips will go a long way with both the criteria listed.

How to avoid feeling underfed

Since you now know how much to eat, let's talk about how to prevent feeling underfed. Believe it or not, both men and women notice this problem, which causes them to overeat. We need to make sure you don't feed underfed to avoid things like breaking a fast too soon or overeating. There is a couple of technique we can provide you with that shall help you with the feeling of underfed.

The first technique we recommend would be eating wholesome, healthy foods which have a lot of fiber in them. Even though you are free to eat whatever you want, it is still not recommended that you eat unhealthily. When you break you're fast, the food you should be eating is high fiber lower carbs and moderate protein. What the fiber will do is help you feel fuller through the day, making you feel less underfed.

An example of this would be to eat more green leafy vegetables, as they will make you feel fuller for a long time. Since we are on the topic of plants, let us talk about vitamins, you need to have micronutrients dense meals when you are fasting. If you are feeling underfed when fasting, the chances are that you are not consuming enough vitamins and minerals, making you feel underfed.

Make sure you are getting your daily mineral intake during your eating window to avoid such adverse effects; you could take a vitamin supplement during your fasting window to obtain your minerals. But don't use the supplement to take care of your vitamin needs, make sure you are eating healthy foods instead of junk food to feel thoroughly fed. Also, drinking water for the whole day is essential. If you are not drinking enough water, then you have a much higher chance of feeling underfed.

Not only will the water help you feel fuller, but it will also help you to get rid of toxins in your body. Water is a must for better fasting experience; another thing which can curb your hunger is coffee. If you drink black coffee during your fast, it will help you control any hunger cravings you might be having which will make you feel less underfed.

One recommendation would be drinking your coffee during the earlier times of the day, instead of later. As drinking coffee then makes you crash pretty hard, which will make you crave more, so make sure you stay away from coffee later during the day. Perhaps consume your coffee earlier in the morning or before your workout works the best, but the main take away would be not to consume junk. Even though fasting allows you to eat whatever you want, it doesn't mean you should, as it can lead you feeling underfed and hungry in the long run. Make sure you are following all these steps to ensure not handling underfed, and as you know, women tend to experience more hunger.

Chapter 7 Can Intermittent Fasting Extend a Woman's Fertility

If intermittent fasting can extend female fertility is a topic that has been asked for a while, but recent studies that were carried out have now shed light on this question. It is no secret that aging causes the reduction of quality and quantity of eggs. The studies were carried out in mice whereby their calorie intake was reduced by 40%. It had significantly improved their egg quality and found out that just a few of their eggs contained abnormal chromosomes when they got to their reproductive years. This is not the same as their counterparts that were allowed to eat as much as they wanted. It is the abnormalities in eggs that usually causes congenital disabilities and raises the risk of having miscarriages. The study further showed that mice that underwent intermittent fasting were able to produce more eggs than the mice that ate as they liked. Restriction of calories also increased the survival of the offspring after birth and also prolonged their reproductive life span. This study concluded that when you manipulate nutrition, you can adjust the signal pathways. Another study was carried out on worms showed that during intermittent fasting, they put reproduction on hold. It helped them to terminate the sex cells that existed to be able to generate healthy eggs. The lifespan of the worms that underwent the process above was greatly extended. Human beings may go through the same process, but tests are yet to be done. The PPAR gamma is the protein that scientists say might do the job of controlling the rate at which ovulation occurs. The studies are also not clear about the amount of calorie restriction that will be needed to turn on such systems in human beings. A lot of fertility problems could be solved if only the identification and manipulation of signaling molecules could be done. This could even extend the reproductive life span of a woman.

Fasting has been said to improve chances of couples that have been trying to conceive through in vitro fertilization but were never successful. Fertility specialists found out that intermittent fasting can alkalize the blood system, removes the synthetic hormones, and cleanse the liver. They also said that when you fast, the body's natural hormone process is rebooted. The calorie intake of people who take the time or find it hard to conceive is usually evaluated. If it is high, with the help of a nutritionist, they are started on intermittent fasting. This will not only get rid of toxins in the patient's body, but it will also help them to get closer to their required Body mass index. Intermittent fasting will cause the rebalancing of hormones, and the liver will metabolize any excess hormones. Fasting will also cause the regeneration of all organs in the body, and issues like inflammation are reduced. It will also boost the immune system and cause the nervous system to be to rest hence making the reproductive system prepared for conception.

In males, intermittent fasting can greatly increase the sperm count from men who suffer from fertility issues. It can also boost the levels of testosterone hormones in men who do not suffer from fertility issues.

-        Intermittent fasting for pregnant women

Intermittent fasting is whereby you voluntarily stay away from food for hours at a time and choose to eat at certain times. Different individuals choose intermittent fasting for various reasons, but the most popular ideas are weight loss and for health benefits. During pregnancy, most women suffer from nausea, and you might start to dislike some foods, usually due to the shifts that happen to hormones that will help in sustaining the pregnancy. When pregnant, the pancreas will grow to produce more insulin. During the first trimester, being nauseous all the time may make it hard for you to overeat on one sitting. Many pregnant women will want to feed on carbohydrates, which will leave you hungry after a short while. It makes intermittent fasting almost impossible due to the number of times you will snack due to hunger. During the second trimester, for most people by now, nausea will have reduced. It can only mean that you can go back to eating a more healthy diet which has fewer carbohydrates and more vegetables and proteins. It will make you stay fuller for longer hours. Fasting while pregnant is not advisable because, during this period, all you need to do is ensure that your micronutrient needs are met. Some pregnant women can go through with fasting without any issue, which is okay. What is not allowed is if you are forcing yourself to fast even though your body is sending hunger signals. The third trimester is where your body's demand for macronutrients is high. When you sleep at night, your body will naturally fast. Therefore, it is not advisable to force your body to go without food because either way, the body typically gains weight. Caution should be applied even though you are advised to eat frequently because overeating junk can cause gestational diabetes, fetal macrosomia, or even preeclampsia. Fasting also is not good when pregnant because the fetus needs nutrients that will support its well-being in the tummy. Fasting is discouraged because when pregnant, the need for protein will be high; hence cannot be met in an 8-hour eating window.

The growing fetus makes the needs for calories and macronutrients high as well and almost impossible to be met in an 8-hour eating window. Your body will also go through some major changes which are hormonally induced because your boy wants to grow a baby. Intermittent fasting should be the last thing on your mind as your total focus should be on the growing fetus.

-        Intermittent fasting for breastfeeding mums.

Extensive research that was carried out on breastfeeding mums showed that short term fasting would not decrease your milk supply. Dehydration is what might cause the decrease in milk. Mothers with babies who are below five months were studied. It was clear that fasting does not affect breast milk or the growth of the baby through what happens is that some essential nutrients in breast milk will reduce. One of the downsides of fasting when breastfeeding is that, you can get dehydrated very fast. This will, in turn, lead to the reduction of breast milk supply and for some mothers it can be extremely difficult to get their milk supply back up. Some of the tips that a breastfeeding mother can use are:

i. Ensure your water intake is high.

For you to maintain milk supply, you need to drink water. This will help to keep you hydrated and reduce hunger pangs.

ii. Consumption of healthy meals.

Eating healthy meals such as vegetables, proteins, and healthy fats such as avocado and nuts will help you go through intermittent fasting smoothly. It will help in the reduction of cravings, and you will only eat healthy foods that will make you feel fuller for longer.

iii. Always start small.

More often than not, after giving birth, all women think about is losing the baby fat. Intermittent fasting may help you shed off a few kilos. Remember, even when in the quest for losing weight, your number one priority should be you and the baby's health. For you to keep your milk supply constant, start small by trying the 12-hour fasting, which is usually the easiest. From there, you can increase your fasting hours gradually.

Be keen and listen to your body.

There is a difference between real hunger, and your body wants to eat. If you are keen enough, you will know whether it's real hunger or if you wish to eat. It is also advisable to pay attention to what triggers your emotions making it easy for you to eat. Make sure you are keen to understand how what you eat affects your body negatively.

iv. Have meal plans.

When on intermittent fasting, it is advisable to have a meal plan. Usually, it is effortless to eat unhealthy foods. Due to hunger, you will eat anything you find, which is less likely to be a balanced diet. Planning will see to it that you eat healthy at all times.

Avoid over-exercising.

Never overdo your exercises. When breastfeeding and on intermittent fasting, it is advisable to stay away from tough workouts. You should increase your intensity as you go because due to starvation, the body does not have a lot of energy. Only mild exercises such as walking and house chores should be done.

67

viii.   Ensure you consume proteins and fiber in all meals.

The advantage of having meals with lots of fiber and proteins is that you will feel fuller for more extended hours, making you avoid overeating or consuming unhealthy foods.

Chapter 8 Autophagy and How Intermittent Fasting Can Improve It

Autophagy is one of the most powerful cleaning processes carried out by the body. Recently, a Japanese scientist Dr. Yoshinori Oshumi won the Nobel peace prize in 2016 for his research on the concept. He found that the body had a very unique ability to purge all the bad elements in the body including the "misformed" proteins, pathogens, and unwanted infections that are harming the body if it senses an acute shortage of energy. This means that if a person is starving, the body would turn off all the bad process in the body and would start using them to produce energy. It would become a highly efficient machine to survive for the longest.

This process can also be used for great advantage as it gives the unique opportunity to get rid of most of the diseases. Even the progression of scariest diseases like cancer can be slowed down with by inducing autophagy. To initiate autophagy, you do not need to do anything extra. You simply need to stop adding anything extra to your body and the process would begin on its own.

Fasting is the only way through which autophagy can begin. Studies have further shown that although long fasts are more effective in initiating autophagy, it can also begin with fasts as small as 12-14 hours every day. This means that by following intermittent fasting you can get the unique advantages of autophagy.

Autophagy is the ultimate solution for most of the diseases in the body. It has the ability to treat diseases and bring longevity. You would feel younger and healthier if your body is going through autophagy. It is the process in which your body is utilizing all the waste products to produce energy and cells. Nothing gets wasted and every resource is put to best use.

The purpose of this chapter is to tell you the ways in which intermittent fasting can help you in getting holistic health. It is not some fad diet that merely helps in losing weight which is only a temporary resort and not even a solution. If your overall health is good, weight management will become effortless and this is the main aim of intermittent fasting.

Intermittent fasting opens the doors of holistic health for you. It makes staying healthy and fit very easy without having to go through the torturous routine of elaborate diets that don't even give you enough to eat. You wouldn't have to keep feeling restricted and desperate through the whole process as eating some of the things becomes a dream. Intermittent fasting will give you great freedom and ease of life. You will simply have to follow some basic rules and the doors of good health will open for you without having to spend large sums of money or time.

Chapter 9 Fasting and Fat Burning and Satiation

There is a rumor circulating that the more you eat, the less hungry you will feel. This means you should eat smaller meals or snacks throughout the day, sometimes as often as 7 times in a day. The concept sounds plausible. If you never truly feel "hungry" because you are constantly eating than the choices, you make regarding what types of food you eat will be better and the amount of food consumed will be lower. Unfortunately, this is not true. Once our body begins a process that is necessary to its survival, like removing waste or drinking water or eating food, it needs to continue until the brain feels satisfied.

Another rumor is that reducing calories or controlling portions can help stop hunger pangs and make you lose weight. While you will most likely lose weight, you will remain hungry. This is because the hormones that tell your brain that it is full and satisfied or still hungry did not get enough juice to balance out. This type of diet is unsustainable for many people, because of these hunger pangs, which results in them losing back all and sometimes more weight than before. It is unsustainable because our bodies are programmed to survive. Hunger is needed for this survival. This means that if it feels that it is always hungry, the hunger triggers will get more and more intense until you finally give in.

This leaves the challenge of how to lose weight and not be hungry all the time. The answer has been in front of us for as long as humanity has been around: fasting.

Fasting removes food from the forefront of your mind and also front-loads your food intake. In addition, it changes your eating schedule so ghrelin, the hunger hormone, is released at different times. Of course, this takes time for your body to adjust, but once it does, the body feels less hungry and is losing weight.

Food at the Front

Eating too many calories will result in weight gain, as evidenced again and again in research, but drastically cutting calories back at meals has been shown to be ineffective at losing weight and keeping it off. This means that on non-fasting days it is important to try to maintain a healthy intake of calories, not gorging yourself on food, but not holding back at breakfast, lunch, and dinner. Those people that eat a standard number of calories on a non-fast day show more satisfaction and less hunger than those that overeat or that try to cut calories back.

When the body feels more satisfied it has balanced itself with the hunger signals, making the hunger survival instinct happy. This means you will lose weight and be able to keep it off. It also means that on fasting days you will begin to feel less hungry as well. After all, as seen above, not eating is better for our instinctual wiring than eating small amounts. For example, if you change jobs and no longer are able to eat lunch at 12 PM and instead need to eat it at 2 PM, your body will feel hungry for a few days at noon but after a while, you will be re-programmed to feel hungry at 2 PM and not 12. The wiring for our rhythms that are based on light, such as sleeping, are more difficult to re-program, but those do not have much to do with hunger. Hunger can be a 24-hour sensation.

As your body goes through it daily flow, hormones and enzymes are released in anticipation of certain activities and transporters of glucose are varied. All of this affects how the body burns energy and loses fat. These responses control your weight, blood sugar, cholesterol, and many other important systems in the body.

As your body goes through it daily flow, hormones and enzymes are released in anticipation of certain activities and transporters of glucose are varied. All of this affects how the body burns energy and loses fat. These responses control your weight, blood sugar, cholesterol, and many other important systems in the body.

Riding the Waves

It has been proven that the hunger hormone is lowest when you first wake up. This is why you may be like many other people and need to wait a bit to eat breakfast. But have you stopped to think about why this is true? Your body has just gone through possibly the longest stretch of time without eating. It would make sense that you would be ravenous when waking, but instead, the body seems satisfied. This is because the body is used to this rhythm and produces less of the hunger hormone.

Next, the body anticipates your schedule. When it senses that it is almost your breakfast, lunch or dinnertime, it releases ghrelin, the hunger hormone. But here is the really interesting thing; the body does not keep producing ghrelin until you eat something. After a bit, the hormone dissipates, regardless of food consumed. It takes about 2 hours for your body to stop responding to the hunger hormone that was released in anticipation of a meal. Think about when you became too busy to eat at your normal time. Did your body eventually "forget" it was hungry? Or did the hunger never even present itself? This is because of the "waves" of hormones being released and then subsiding.

Research has shown that throughout a 24-hour day, fasting or non-fasting, ghrelin is released at the same levels. This means that you are not hungrier on fasting days, but rather you are the same. This means that as your body becomes conditioned to eating on a different schedule, you will become less hungry, not more. When you are less hungry, you are less likely to eat more, and less likely to gain weight. But you are more likely to lose it!

Women do show a markedly more intense and faster change to ghrelin during a fasting state. This means women will adjust faster to a new eating pattern than men. To account for this, women may be more suitable to do a one-on-one-off fast while men may benefit from a three-on- four-off type of fast to see similar results. When you fast, whether you are a man or woman, you can expect your ghrelin levels to drop. You can expect your body to send you messages that you are less hungry and more satisfied. You can also expect to not be "able" or do not desire to eat as much as you used to. You will feel fuller faster. You may also no longer crave the treats you used to turn to on a regular basis. This demonstrates the biological and mental changes happening in your body.

Overall, this means that fasting can and does make you feel less hungry and lose weight after your body adjusts to the new rhythm. Your body will adjust the release of ghrelin when you train it to and you can ride out the waves of hunger as they pass without turning into a ravenous animal. Fasting is truly one of the most sustainable and effective methods for losing and keeping weight off!

Chapter 10 The Science of Hunger

Inside your brain, there is a pathway that is programmed for your love of food, specifically the really "good" foods. This pathway is not something you were born with, but it was developed over time. The neurochemical, sensory and metabolic reactions fired the minute you tasted that first "treat." The pleasure center in your brain, the mesolimbic area, is what became engaged. Digestive acids were secreted when your stomach received the signal from the vagus nerve.

Insulin began being pumped out by the pancreas. The increase in sugar, fat, and starch are accommodated by increased liver production. During this whole process, your brain simply remembers that whatever it was that you just ate was good. This begins a lasting impression of that particular food.

Your relationship with food as a human is difficult. Many of your body's systems occur automatically, such as your endocrine, circulatory, and respiratory systems. Eating is distinctive because it is completely voluntary and critical to your life. This is the reason for the intense desire for food that you feel. This is a problem now because, instead of the age-old problem of not having enough to eat, we now face the issue of having too much. Your body is not programmed to handle the unrestrained options that are available to your uncontrolled appetite.

Our appetite often drives our behavior, so it is important to learn how to control it. This control has been difficult to pinpoint because it is an incredibly complex process. All the senses, the chemistry of the brain and gut, and even psychology are involved. This is what science is still working to understand. Part of this research includes looking to the past to decipher how our ancestors controlled their hunger and how we can use this to our advantage. Fasting is part of this research.

For your ancestors, the state of your weight is what they sought after. These ancestors did not know where their next meal was coming from and often faced dangerous risks while trying to get something to eat. For example, sampling crops that they did not know or hunting animals for meat endangered their lives almost daily. This means that when they did have good food they needed to eat as much as possible. Human bodies are programmed to eat a lot when it is available and especially eat fat-filled food. There is a reason your body takes several minutes to recognize that it is full after eating a meal. After 20 minutes your body will recognize it is still hungry, full, or over full. This served your ancestors well because they could eat a lot before their body shut them off, but it is not so helpful now.

Your body does work internally to regulate itself. You're eating habits are established through your routine. When you consume meals or snacks at certain times of the day on a regular basis your body begins to anticipate eating and sends a hunger signal through a hormone named ghrelin. This hormone is created in the gut and is produced by our dietary schedule and even possibly the smell or sight of food. It creates the sensation of an empty stomach that the brain interprets as feeling hungry. In the brain, the hypothalamus, which is the director of the metabolism, the midbrain's mesolimbic center, which is the pleasure center, and the hindbrain, which governs unconscious procedures, are all hit by the production of ghrelin. This is why the brain listens to the signal from the gut.

There is a balance to the production of ghrelin and the signal it sends to the brain. This counter-balance begins in the upper intestine and stomach. This is a physical response to becoming full. The tension and stretching of the organs send a signal after time to the brain. This sensation includes three more items that signal the brain. CCK, or cholecystokinin, is a peptide from the upper intestine. It tells the brain you are satisfied and to stop eating. This only lasts a short time compared to ghrelin. What arrives in the brain after CCK are GLP-1 and PYY, hormones that reinforce the signal to stop. These hormones come from the lower gut and some of it stays behind to also talk to the stomach. These hormones let the stomach know it needs to pause sending food to the digestive tract until it has processed what is already there. GLP-1 also alerts the pancreas to send more insulin out to help absorb the sugar from the foods ingested and then store them in the fat for later energy.

If the balance between these two systems becomes off-kilter and you are still eating too much and gaining weight, there is another natural regulator: leptin. Your body's fat produces this hormone that stifles the appetite. The more the hormone is produced is proportional to the fat tissue in the body. Once the hormone hits the bloodstream, it travels to the brain's hypothalamus and seeks a partnership with neuropeptides that stimulate the appetite. This partnership results in the neuropeptides being slightly stifled. Ideally, this means that the more weight you have the more leptin you have to help control appetite.

The reason these internal forces do not always self-regulate your body is that there are approximately twenty-four other peptides and hormones that control the appetite. This means that changing just one or two hormones or levels will not result in a large change in appetite and weight. It truly does require a complete overhaul of the system.

Additional research into some of the complex receptors in the brain that create gateways for appetite signals is underway. MC-3 and MC-4 are the two currently most interesting pathways. MC-4 can malfunction, not allowing the "correct" signals to be interpreted in the brain, and MC- 3 can also become dysfunctional and not allow the body to balance itself. Other research is being conducted regarding the "addiction" to eating and the chemical responses our brains and bodies go through when eating or abstaining.

Chapter 11 Secret Techniques for Feasting on Your Favorite Foods

So, you may be thinking by this point, "Wait, I go hours, even days, without food?" Well, sort of. Maybe. When you are in a fasting period, you will have spans of time when you will decide if you want to consume nothing but non-caloric beverages, such as coffee, tea, and water, or if you want to stick to a plan that has minor or no caloric intake from foods. The reason for this is to prevent the body's insulin response from being active. You want the body to need to pull from the fat storage in your body for energy and fuel, not burn up what you are putting into it.

When you are breaking your fast and have a period of freedom in what and when you can eat, keep in mind that you need to ease in slowly. It is not the best idea to load up on carbs in your first meal after a fasting period. Doing this would send your insulin response system into "overdrive" right after a dormant period. Instead, try reaching for vegetables and fresh fruits. If you desire carbs, try a small serving of whole-grain pasta. Stay away from slices of bread and heavy carbohydrates for the first meal after a fast. This advice is contrary to people who are intensifying their workout during a fasting period. If this is the case for you, then a carb-heavy meal is necessary and your body will use those incoming fuel sources fast. It is also ill-advised to eat a very spicy meal right after fasting. This can cause indigestion and inflammation.

But these suggestions are just that: suggestions. If you have an iron stomach and are fine with spicy foods, then by all means, enjoy a good "hot" meal after your fast. You can still enjoy all your favorite foods while intermittent fasting, just mindfully on the days when you break your fast. Remember, if you are looking to lose weight, your calories cannot be greater than your calories out. This means if you overeat on non-fasting days, also called "feasting" days, you will negate the progress you made during the fast. Instead, choose the foods you want to enjoy in relation to that calorie goal for the rest of the day.

Another common question or concern is how often a person can eat during a "feasting" day. This is dependent on your preferences and your intermittent fasting plan. If you only have 8 hours to eat in, you can choose to eat all your calories in two large meals or three small meals, or just in snacking on healthy foods throughout the day.

If you are doing a 24-hour fast and will not have another meal until dinnertime, you may eat a large dinner with a small snack later in the evening, but not much else during that day. You do not need to adhere to a "standard" meal plan with breakfast, lunch, and dinner occurring at specific times of the day. Instead, consider what times of the day you have to dedicate to eating well and what you prefer to do. Some people like the "visual" of "skipping" breakfast for his or her fasting, meaning they will not eat breakfast foods that day, but instead will eat a good lunch and dinner. Others will only count the hours of the fast and eat breakfast when the fast is broken, then adjust their meal times from there.

A word of caution for those considering the snacking option: be prepared with what you will "snack" on during your fasting days. Pre-packaged snacks tend to be heavy with carbs and calories, having little nutritional benefit. Preparing healthy meals are often more beneficial to your overall goals, but it requires more time on a feast day. If you want to snack throughout your day, plan ahead with healthy grab-and-go options you know will satisfy your hunger, calorie goals, and nutritional needs.

Always keep in mind that breaking your fast early or re-adjusting your needs throughout the process is acceptable and encouraged. This is supposed to be a sustainable meal planning process that fits into your life. If you feel, at hour 22, that you need to eat now or you will end up with a 48-hour fast because of your schedule, then eat! In addition, if you are in your first two weeks of adopting an intermittent fasting plan, and you find that one day is plenty and you do not want to do a full second day this week, take the day off or cut the fast shorter. Keep in mind, though, that the body requires about 13 hours for it to clear out remaining glucose and begin burning body fat. If you break your fast before 13 hours, you could be preventing your body from tapping into that backup energy storeroom. If you can, try to make it to 14 hours, if possible, but again, adjust as needed for your life. Another mental game you can play with yourself during this process is to see if you can extend the fasting period safely. For example, if you are doing a 16/8, what if you fasted for 17, giving yourself a window of 7 hours to eat your calories for the day? Trying to think about extending, rather than shortening, can make the time commitment not feel as stressed.

If you are starting off this process slowly and are cutting back on calories, stay within your selected calorie intake for the "fasting" day and then release the pressure of counting calories on the "feasting" day. Yes, it may take you longer to see results because you may be eating over your recommended calorie limit for your age and weight, but the idea is to give you the habit of fasting and then feasting. From there, you can begin to cut out food altogether during a fasting day or can begin counting calories on feasting days. It is up to you how you want to advance your intermittent fasting, so do not feel boxed into counting and restricting. Start with developing the habit first, and then move in the direction that makes the most sense for you.

Consider your favorite foods now. What are the foods that you love to go for when you treat yourself or want to indulge? These are foods you can still enjoy and savor when following an intermittent fasting plan. The caveat is that now you enjoy them on your feasting days or time window. If you are trying to lose weight and want results faster, take a look at the number of calories in these treats. How many treats can you eat within your feasting day or time frame without going over the calorie limit? For example, most women should stay below a 1,800 calorie day. If you know that your favorite ice cream has 500 calories per serving, you could only eat 3 servings of that ice cream, leaving 300 calories for other foods (hopefully with a nutritional content!). You may not want to dedicate all those calories on your feasting day to that ice cream, but what if you only had one scoop? What could you spend the rest of the 1,300 calories on? It could even be feasible to consider a half scoop of the ice cream, leaving you even more calories to allocate to other foods during the feasting time. If you love hamburgers, look at how many calories it contains and decide if you want the full burger or half of it. The same goes with a side of fries. Do you really need to eat the large portion or will you be happy with the small size and leaving more calories for something else later?

The wonderful thing about intermittent fasting is that you do not need to remove your favorite indulgences from your life forever. You are just selecting a specific time you will eat them, and if you want to go further with it, you will decide how much of it you want to eat during that time. You get to choose your own goals, time frame, and rules. As long as you are patient with the process, you can go as slow into the intermittent fasting plan as you want to. This is a great example of starting in slowly, but your expectations need to match the speed. A slow start means a slow result. There is nothing wrong with that, in fact, it is a great place to be, but remember that as you measure your waist or step on the scale in the morning after a "fast" day. For those looking to lose weight more quickly, consider a more structured and restrictive approach while still falling within the appropriate guidelines. An alternate-day intermittent fast for two weeks with a healthy calorie limit on "feast" days can help you jumpstart your body's fat-burning process, but it requires a focused and committed approach. You may also not be able to enjoy many of your favorite foods during this two-week time frame. It is a tradeoff for speed, but it does not mean you have to say goodbye to chips, chocolate, or your other favorite foods for a long time and definitely not forever!

Below is a list of some of the more common "favorite foods" and their common calorie range. You can use this as a foundation for planning purposes. Explore what your favorite brands or foods are on your own to create your personal, customized favorite foods list to be more exact. You can follow the same format and design a list to reference when you need and want to. Keep in mind, this is a helpful tool for those that are restricting calories to a healthy range on the days that food is consumed or "feasting" days. This is not relevant to you if you are only focusing on caloric intake on fasting days. It is also not relevant for you if you do not want it to be! Choose to follow this or not, consume as much of your favorite foods on a feasting day as you want or find a limit. It is your call. And again, you can always start off slow, and then move into this phase of intermittent fasting.

Favorite Food and Drink	Common Calorie Range
Bagel	289
Beer, regular	153
Chocolate chip cookie	59
Soda, one cup	136
Graham cracker	59
Vanilla ice cream	145
Burger patty, no bun or toppings	193
Hot dog, no bun or toppings	137
Jelly donut	289
Ketchup, 1 tablespoon	15

Oatmeal, plain	147
Peanut butter, 2 tablespoons	180
Pepperoni pizza, one slice	298
Baked potato, no toppings	161
Salted potato chips, 1 ounce	155
Salted hard pretzels, 1 ounce	108
Ranch dressing, 2 tablespoons	146
Red wine, 5 ounces	123
White rice, 1 cup	205
Salsa, 4 ounces	35
Plain spaghetti, 4 ounces	221
Spaghetti sauce, 1 cup	92

White wine, 5 ounces	121
Chocolate-frosted vanilla cake, 1 piece	243
Bacon, 2 pieces	250
Sausage, pork, 2 pieces	250-290
Cream cheese	200
Chewing gum, 1 piece	9
Chocolate	200
Popcorn	150
White sugar, 1 teaspoon	20
Chik-Fil-A Waffle Fry, medium	360
Chik-Fil-A chicken sandwich	440
McDonald's french fries, medium	340

McDonald's hamburger	250
McDonald's chicken nuggets, 4 count	270
Taco Bell cheesy gordita crunch with shredded beef	500
Taco Bell nachos	310
Wendy's natural cut fries	228
Wendy's homestyle chicken sandwich	520
Wendy's Junior cheeseburger	280
Bread, white, 1 slice	96
Fried fish fingers or fish sticks, 1 piece	50
Lunch meats	300
Canned tuna, in water	100

Apple, 1	44
Banana, 1	107
Baked beans	170
Carrots	16
Celery	5
Dates	100
Olives	50
Orange	40
Peach	35
Pear	45
Pineapple	40
Plum	30
Strawberry, 1 large	10
Corn on the cob	70

Tomato	30
Cheese slice, 1 ounce	110
Cottage cheese	49
Egg, 1	90
Whole milk, 1 cup	175
Omelet with cheese	300
Plain yogurt	90
Butter, 1 tablespoon	112
Honey, 1 tablespoon	42
Jelly, 1 tablespoon	38
Margarine, 1 tablespoon	50
Avocado	150

Chapter 12 Diet, Nutrition, Exercise, Rest

An understanding of the kind of foods, and what you will gain in nutrition are all part of the fasting plan. In addition, an exercise regimen, along with the types of exercises that are the most beneficial, will be covered. Finally, getting sufficient rest to allow the program to do what you want it to do – lose weight, improve your health and mental clarity will round out the plan.

As you have already read, intermittent fasting does not require calorie counting, pills or potions, and does not create eating disorders. What it does is allow you to fast during a certain pre-determined window of time and then "break" the fast by eating for a period of time.

But, before you even get to that point, you need to do the one thing that will ascertain if fasting is the right thing for you to do and that consults with your health professional. People who have Type 1 diabetes, women who are pregnant or lactating should not take on intermittent fasting. Their bodies need around-the-clock balance of foods and nutrients. Additionally, anyone who has been diagnosed with a binge-eating disorder will tend to overeat during their eating window, thus not making intermittent fasting a good program for them to follow. Their binging and overeating will defeat the purpose of fasting to lose weight. (Cole, n.d.)

Diet and Nutrition

There are many facets to the diet. Not only what you should eat, but why you should eat them is important to understand. A major ingredient in the fast is to eat not just what's low in calorie, but what will give your body the most nutrition it needs. Once you begin to incorporate the suggested foods, you'll probably find yourself feeling fuller for longer periods. Keep the meals you eat as simple as possible and don't forget that snacks are allowed as well. It's not about calorie counting; it's about eating the right foods to promote weight loss and healthy eating.

How Intermittent Fasting Affects Our Body

Cells, Hormones, and Genes Change Their Function

Your body goes through a number of different changes when you don't eat and are in a fasted state. Your body begins important cellular repair procedures and the hormone levels to make stored fat accessible changes.

Insulin levels – blood levels of insulin drop radically, enabling fat burning.

Cellular Repair -The removal of waste material from cells that is important in cellular repair, known as autophagy.

Gene Expression – beneficial in several molecules and genes that are related to the protection against disease and longevity.

HGH (human growth hormone) – a growth hormone, blood levels may increase as much as five times higher than normal. These higher levels of HGH allows for muscle gain and fat burning, along with numerous other benefits. (Gunnars BSc, 2016)

Eating the Wrong Foods Can Counter the Benefits

Intermittent Fasting is not considered a diet, it's an eating pattern. Correctly implemented, it promotes reducing blood sugar, healthy brain function, and weight loss and maintenance. Supposedly, the best part is that when you can eat, it can be what you want to eat over the amount of time allotted during the day.

That last line is not exactly true. If you practice intermittent fasting but overeat at your meal times, you're defeating the whole purpose of the practice.

Eating the right foods in order to gain the benefits of the plan, the suggestion is to eat the right foods that provide the nutrients your body needs to carry you through your non-eating periods.

Since intermittent fasting works on the idea of calorie restriction and you fast for 24 hours but eat twice the amount of food than you normally would during the following 24 hour period, then the fast was negated. The quality of what you consume during your eating periods is important. (Shulman, 2018)

Getting all of your nutrition from fewer meals is the goal. You don't want to waste the space on your plate with foods that have zero or very little nutrients. The foods that you can get your vitamins, minerals, and nutrients are below:

Important Food Groups for Nutrition

In order to derive as much nutrition from the foods that will sustain you during your fasting period, you should be eating full and satisfying meals laden with lean animal proteins, whole grains, vegetables, and berries.

What Nutrition You Get from Lean Protein *(Food Network, n.d.)*

Eggs – One egg offers just 70 calories and 6 grams of protein. Most of the protein is in egg whites, so add extra egg whites. Pack one to eat as a snack or add a hard-boiled egg to a salad.

Skinless turkey or chicken – The leanest choice is white meat. You can also consider dark meat. 25 grams of protein, selenium, and B vitamins can be found in chicken and turkey.

Ground Beef - 90% (or leaner) – It is a good protein source. Zinc, iron, vitamin B, and 22 grams of protein can be found in just 3 ounces of lean beef.

Beans and Lentils – these should be eaten as much as possible. They give you 9 grams of protein per half cup and are a good source of fiber, folate which is good for the heart, and iron.

Low and Nonfat Dairy - dairy products are good sources of lean protein such as ricotta cheese, yogurt, cottage cheese, and milk. You can have smoothies for breakfast that have fruits and skim milk or whole grain toast with honey pumpkin seeds, lemon zest, and ricotta. (Food Network, n.d.)

Fish and Shellfish - It is recommended by the (American Heart Association) to eat every week at least two servings of 3.5 ounces. Keep a few cans of Alaskan salmon or light tuna on hand to include in a salad or make a sandwich.

Pork Loin – loin chops, sirloin roast, and pork tenderloin are lean cuts of pork. In just three-ounce serving, you can get B vitamins and 23 grams of protein.

Tofu and Other Soy Foods – One of the highest vegetarian sources of protein is soy. ½ cup provides 8-10 grams of protein and 1 cup of edamame provides 8 grams of fiber and 17 grams of protein.

Nuts, Nut Butters, and Seeds – A study by Harvard researchers found that nuts are connected to weight loss. They are fiber-filled and provide healthy fats. Peanut or almond butter is great on toast. Mix sunflower and pumpkin seed with dried fruit for a snack.

Healthy Carbohydrates *(Food Network, n.d.)*

Sweet Potatoes – the orange color is part of what makes the sweet potato so healthy. They contain vitamin A's forerunner, beta-carotene, which is vital for your immune system and vision.

Legumes – beans and lentils have complex carbs, fiber, and protein. These foods fill you up.

Milk – milk, yogurt, cottage cheese, and other dairy products contain a type of sugar, lactose. Milk provides sodium and protein. When these three components are combined, it can be a good drink after working out.

Fruit – If you love sweets, you can eat fruits. The sweetness of the fruit comes from fructose. It is a balance of minerals, vitamins, phytochemicals, water, and fiber. Sweeter fruits like bananas and mangoes are a great source of energy which low-carb diets avoid.

Popcorn – believe it or not, popcorn has a high amount of antioxidants and is considered as a whole grain. 3 ½ cups can be had from a 1-ounce serving. If air popped, that would give you 4 grams of fiber and 110 calories.

Potatoes – potatoes are an excellent source of potassium and vitamin C, along with 4 grams fiber found in a medium potato. They are in the glycemic index, but you never eat them alone. They get topped with cheese, mashed with milk, and baked in the oven, gives you a toasty fiber-rich skin to eat. These additives prevent your blood sugar from rising and bring the glycemic index down.

Whole grains – there are two that you are already familiar with – whole grain bread and pasta, but get acquainted with other unprocessed grains – rye, oats, quinoa, and farro for additional health benefits.

An example of a satisfying satiating meal could be wild rice, with roasted salmon or baked white fish with a side of veggies and an avocado with a dash of olive oil, and for dessert, a small bowl of berries. With this type of meal, you get enormous amounts of nutrition and feel strong and energized the next morning. (Shulman, 2018)

Does Intermittent Fasting and Exercise go together?

So, how do you fast and incorporate exercise? Do you think you'll be too tired? How is intermittent fasting affecting your energy level? The key to exercise is the timing of when you do (or don't) eat that can impact your workout.

Exercising shows that when you are in the fasted state, fat oxidation and lipolysis are both increased. Also, the abdominal region receives blood flow. Belly fat is not easy to lose because of impaired blood flow. Fasting training can help in overcoming this.

Certified sports nutritionist and former exercise science professor Gabrielle Fundaro, Ph.D. says this about the type of exercise you're going to get into, "When you're doing 30 minutes of cardio, that's fine to do fasting, but if you're doing cardio for a much longer period, your body is going to rely on stored glycogen – which is sugar used for energy for intensive activities – so your workout and your performance may not be as good. (Laurence, Emily, 2018)

In other words, a short workout session when you fasted will be a lot better than a longer, more intense workout. A good tip would be to eat a small meal or snack between three hours and 20 minutes before your workout so you have glycogen ready to fuel the body. The snack can be an apple with nut butter or a piece of toast with peanut butter. If you want to avoid the carbs, you can eat yogurt with nuts.

Dr. Fundaro advises that if you decide to do weight training, it's advised to do so during your eating window. This is important because if you do weight training while in the fasted state, you can damage the muscle tissue. After you finish your workout, any meal you have should include a good amount of protein to rebuild muscle.

Go for a high-intensity workout after eating

Generally, if you schedule any moderate to intense workout sessions to your last meal, the better. You'll still have leftover carbs available to energize your workout and the risk of low blood sugar will be reduced. (Fetters, 2016)

Eat High Protein Meals

If you are looking to build muscle, you'll need to eat before and after a high-intensity workout and, you need to eat. A pre-workout snack can help give you fuel, consuming protein is vital to muscle synthesis throughout the day and immediately after your strength workout. That is when your muscles are hungering for amino acids to allow them to repair themselves and grow. (Fetters, 2016)

Listen to your body. Eat if you're hungry, either before or after your workout or at times when it's been weeks since you worked out. (Laurence, Emily, 2018)

Rest

This is extremely important to the success of your intermittent fasting program. It is said that when you fast, you have more energy and that your sleep pattern improves.

When your sleep is shortened, there is a decrease of leptin and increase of ghrelin. This means you will feel hunger more acutely. Research has found that if you get six hours of sleep every night for two weeks, your physical and mental functioning diminishes to the equivalent as if you remained awake for a straight 48 hours.

We sleep better when we turn off our laptops, tablets, and phones and spend time relaxing before bed, our digestive system needs to relax and wind down as well before we are ready for sleep.

Intermittent fasting plays a part in how much better we sleep and how much more we derive from our sleep. We fall asleep more rapidly and sleep more soundly through the night. What we get is more restful sleep. (Weingus, Leigh, n.d.)

Eating a healthy diet of protein, whole grains, and healthy fats will provide the nutrients your body will need to carry you through your periods of fast.

Studies have shown that intermittent fasting improves several risk factors such as heart disease, blood pressure, triglycerides, inflammatory markers, and cholesterol levels.

Exercise is beneficial as well but should be less strenuous when you're fasting. Gentle stretching or yoga will be better for you during your fast window.

In order to benefit from intermittent fasting, your body needs a sufficient amount of rest as well in order to prevent the onset of extreme hunger.

As you learn more about intermittent fasting, you'll understand how the food you consume during your eating window will supply the nutrition your body needs to maintain brain capacity, the balance of insulin levels, hormone growth, and cellular repair. All important functions of a healthy life.

Chapter 13 Common Mistakes to Avoid

Intermittent Fasting is a great process that can bring exemplary health effects. However, any process can only work efficiently if its execution is right and silly mistakes are not done in the execution.

This chapter will explain some of the common mistakes people make while following intermittent fasting. This chapter will focus on the basic mistakes that we make casually but which can harm our weight loss goals as well as health goals drastically.

Pay Attention to Macronutrients

This is one of the most important things to remember. The people who are suffering from obesity simply wants to get rid of this malice. They are ready to barter anything for it. They dream of a slender figure as the ultimate goal and this is where they become susceptible to make some of the most fatal mistakes.

Intermittent fasting or any form of dieting or calorie restrictive routine would put certain restrictions on you. Intermittent fasting doesn't put a cap on the amount of food you can eat or its type. However, that doesn't mean you can eat a lot. In most cases, you will have only 7-8 hours in reality to eat anything that you want. Missing that meal may mean that you'll have to go without food till the next meal. Therefore, the amount of food you can eat gets limited.

Other calorie restrictive routines put an explicit cap on the amount and type of food you can have. These things have a profound impact on your health. You may experience weight loss but that doesn't mean that you are getting healthy.

Your body can only get healthy when it is getting all the macro and micronutrients in the right quantity. It also needs vitamins and minerals. Getting all that while consuming limited calories can be difficult. If you don't pay proper attention here, you will end up with nutrient deficiencies.

You may get a slender frame but you will be battling with more problems than you started with.

The best way to counter this problem is to have a properly balanced diet. Intermittent fasting allows you a proper chance to do so as it doesn't put restrictions on quantity and types of food items you can have.

The best way to pass this trick with qualifying marks is to have a very balanced meal. Your meals should be high in fat, moderate in protein and low in carbs.

Before you begin to question the credibility of the suggestion, I would like to clarify some misconceptions:

Fat is not bad

There is a popular misconception that eating fat is bad. Fat is the building block of life. It plays a number of important roles in our life. Our body can not function without fat. Fat, in general, is not bad. Trans fat or the poor quality fat that we get in processed food is bad. Fat in itself is a form of compact energy. Our body doesn't classify food as fat, protein, or cholesterol. Everything that you eat gets processed and is broken down as calories. This means that fat would also get converted to glucose, and so would happen with carbs. The benefit of eating fat is that you will be able to get more calories in a single meal in comparison to carbs.

Fat is very compact in nature and has almost double the number of calories per gram when compared to carbs. So if you get 8 calories per gram of carbs you'll get 16 from fat. Protein is also heavier and has more calories than carbs. This means that if you consume a high fat – low carb diet, you can get more calories. It also means that even if you have fewer meals in a day, you will not get energy deficient.

Fat should be consumed in greater quantities. You should select high-quality fat. The same goes for protein. You can get protein from animals and cereals and it would help you in muscle building and staying fit. The biggest advantage of having a high-fat, moderate protein, low carb diet is that it doesn't make you feel hungry very often. Fat and protein content in your meals would help you in transitioning from one meal to the other easily without facing the need to have snacks.

Fat and protein-rich diets also contain a lot of minerals and vitamins. However, the highest part of minerals and vitamins and fiber should be obtained from carbs. You should consume a lot of leafy green vegetables, salads, whole grain foods. Leafy greens are bulky and but they do not weigh much. They don't add too many calories to your system but they provide most of the vitamins, minerals, phytonutrients, antioxidants and trace minerals required by your body. You can have leafy green vegetables as much as you want without worrying about calories. They are rich in fiber and hence keep your digestive system healthy and improve your immunity as well.

This is a part that you should never undermine in your pursuit to have a slender figure. If you ignore your health, the weight would come back faster than you can lose it. It will also have a very adverse impact on your health.

You must always remember that you need to be healthy to fight weight and it isn't the other way around. The people who lose their weight drastically without a solid base are called sick and not healthy.

You must never forget the macronutrients in your meal as they would become the pillars of your health.

Don't Get Greedy in the Feasting Windows

Food has its own temptation. It looks like the most alluring thing in the world when you have been deprived of it for a long time. This would happen with you too. But, it is important that you don't get greedy at such times and lose control. It is very important that you get off your fasting windows in a proper manner.

The biggest mistake people make is they eat a lot after breaking their fast. This can cause several problems and poor digestion is one among them. In the fasting state, the gut gets to stay away from food for extended periods and hence it can get a bit dry. Stuffing it with heavy food can cause problems. The best way to begin the day is to start with liquid food and then transition to semi-solid and solids.

You should also mind the quantity of food that you eat. Our brain takes much longer to understand the leptin signals that you are full. By the time your brain tells you that you are full, you would have already overeaten. The best way out is to either eat slowly as this would give your brain the time to assess your satiety levels. You can also stop eating when you feel that you are 80% full. Generally, by this time you would have eaten your fill. If you want to test this, you can wait for sometime after feeling 80% full and you'd find that you are no longer feeling hungry. It happens as the fat cells are able to properly communicate to the brain that it doesn't need to eat anymore.

Don't Try to Rush the Process

Slow and steady wins the race. This is an adage we all have heard but most of us fail to believe. We want quick results and for that, we are ready to make the jumps. However, this is not how the body works. Your body makes the transition very slowly. It needs the time to adjust to any kind of change positive or negative and the same would happen even in case of intermittent fasting.

If you want to succeed with the process you must ensure that you stick to every stage for some time. You must give your body the required time to adjust. There would be decades old habits that would need to change and it can be difficult for your body at times. If you want your body to react favorably to the change, you must not rush the process.

Fasting in men and women is completely different. Men have a very rugged system and it doesn't get affected by a bit extended fasting schedule. However, it isn't the case with women. If you try to jerk your system a bit harder, it can affect your health adversely. Your hormonal system may go for a spin and it may take very long for it to normalize. A woman's body reacts very differently to stress signals and hence caution and patience are essential.

Start with the easiest process and give your body the time to adjust to the small breaks. Once it gets used to a certain amount of brake, try to extend it a bit slowly. Don't do anything very fast. Always go step by step and you will get your goal easily and without unnecessary difficulties.

Perseverance is the Key

Impatience is a big problem in people battling with weight. There is no fault of theirs as they are already under great pressure. Most people trying to lose weight have already faced disappointment with other weight loss measures and hence they want to see the results fast to believe them. They are not ready to wait very long to get the results.

This is a point where problems can occur. Intermittent fasting is not any wonder-process. It is a wonderful process but it doesn't work by magic. It tries to correct the problems that may have reached their current state of development in decades at least.

It would take some time for the results to come. You will have to work patiently and not lose hope while the results come. If you quit in between, you wouldn't be able to know if you were making any progress or not. It isn't a process that works overnight. It would require you to take the leap of faith and invest your time and energy into it.

Don't Frame Unrealistic Expectations

We all like to dream big and that is a good thing. However, we must also remain grounded in reality. This will help in accepting the facts and save a lot of disappointments. Many times we are so engrossed with the imaginary expectations that we fail to recognize the gifts we get. If weight loss is your goal then think of the amount of time you are ready to devote, the lengths to which you can go for it and the medical conditions you are facing. Without considering all these facts, expecting a complete makeover would be absurd. If you have made such expectations then you will not even be able to enjoy the weight loss you are observing. Your expectations would overshadow the results. It is important that you remain realistic.

Properly Manage Your Fasting Time

It isn't unusual for some people to mismanage their time. Most of us do it in our daily lives. However, poor management of the fasting time can be a cause of great distress for you. It can make your weight loss journey difficult and painful. You cannot remain thinking about food all the while you are in the fasted state. This would create problems for you and your gut would also remain confused.

The best way to manage the fasting time is to keep yourself busy. The last leg of your fasting window should always be planned in such a way that you remain aptly engaged. The idler you are the higher are the chances that you'll only think about food.

Engaging in heavy physical activity is one of the best ways to put off hunger. The hunger in today's age is a highly psychological phenomenon. Our bodies have ample energy stores to run without food for months. It is our mind that is always drawing us towards food. You only need to stall it for a few hours.

Walking, running, laughing, talking to friends, engaging in serious discussions are some of the ways through which we can stall hunger and remain unaffected.

These are some of the common mistakes that we make and which can mar the results we get. Intermittent fasting is a very simple and easy way to lose weight. It doesn't require much of your time and effort. You only need to make up your mind once and bring it into your life. Even if you are following any other weight loss measure, intermittent fasting can still fit into your lifestyle.

Chapter 14 Tips and Tricks

Before we send you on your way to your new healthy lifestyle, there are a few important tips and tricks for you to learn and keep up your sleeve. In the beginning, it always seems easy to begin a new diet. You have this new found motivation and energy to change your life. But, what happens when that energy burns out in a few weeks? By knowing some tips and tricks about the plant-based diet, these will keep you going when times get rough!

Getting Started on a Plant-based Diet

1. Find Your Motivation

Truly, I cannot express the importance of this enough! If you are here in this book, there was probably something drastic that made you want to make a major change. This reason is your why and what you should set your goals around. Whether you are looking for mental clarity, more energy, or helping a disease, always try to remember why you are starting this lifestyle in the first place. For bonus points, write down your why on a sheet of paper so that you can look at it when you need added motivation.

2. Remember to Eat

It will be important that you remember to eat more than you are used to. Luckily on a plant-based diet, you can say goodbye to counting calories. Now, you can fill up on salad, fruit, quinoa, beans, and even baked potatoes to your heart's content! The whole point of this diet is to live off the good food, and over time, the body adjusts to the volume of food. After a while, you will learn to rely on your satiety cues and natural hunger.

3. Prepare Food

As you start a plant-based diet, I encourage you to take a stroll through your kitchen. In the beginning, you will begin to recognize the foods that may not be as beneficial to you as a whole food. I suggest you toss these foods or give them away, so you keep yourself out of temptations reach. Instead, fill your fridge and pantry with healthy foods such as beans, rice, and potatoes! This way when you get cravings for unhealthy foods, there won't be any in your house!

4. Take it Gentle

Switching over to a plant-based diet does not need to happen overnight! Instead, I suggest taking a gentler approach and slowly switch your diet to become more plant-based. If you make sudden changes, you could potentially feel restricted and ultimately cheat yourself out of your amazing diet. An example would be to use avocado instead of butter! While it is a change, it will take some time to get used to. As you increase the healthy plant-based ingredients in your life, you will slowly eliminate the bad stuff.

5. One Meal at a Time

There are no rules saying that being plant-based needs to be a now or never type of deal. Instead, try switching one meal at a time to be more plant-based. One of the easier meals, I have found, is breakfast! Instead of your normal milk and cereal, give oatmeal with your favorite fruit a try! There is also delicious avocado toast or breakfast potatoes! I highly suggest trying some of the recipes provided in this book to help you get started! Slowly, you can switch all of your meals to being plant-based, and soon it won't even be a second thought.

6. Find Good People

Typically, it is easier to go through changes when you have company to share your struggles and successes with. It is a fantastic idea to form a support group so you can reach out for help and inspire others. I suggest checking out internet forums or even Facebook groups for you to connect with. Just remember that you are never alone on this journey!

7. Keep it Fun

Switching to a plant-based diet is not meant to be a form of torture. I hope that eventually, you learn to enjoy your food choices and perhaps even look forward to it. Luckily with modern technology, you have recipes at your fingertips. There are always new foods to try and recipes to give a shot. A good way to keep your diet fun is to have an adventurous side. The next time you visit the grocery store, I challenge you to choose out a fruit or vegetable that you have never heard of before. When you have made your selection, use the internet to find ideas on how to cook this item. You may be surprised at what you learn about food and about yourself!

8. Commit

As you begin the plant-based diet, the best thing you can do is make the commitment to yourself. There are a number of reasons people begin the plant-based diet. Why are you here? Why do you feel a plant-based diet can change your life? At the end of the day, it does not matter what anyone else thinks. If you want to make this commitment to yourself, you make this commitment! It is time to take your health into your own hands. You are the only one who can make health decisions for yourself, make sure those decisions are the best ones possible. You owe yourself that much.

Plant-based on a Budget

One major excuse individuals use not to eat healthily is that they feel eating healthy can be too expensive. The trick here is to make smart choices. There are plenty of ways to strip the diet down to the basics; whole foods can actually be easily affordable for just about anyone! All you need is some knowledge about whole foods, and you will be able to fit all of your nutrients into your budget with ease!

9. Stay Home!

This seems like a given but eating at home instead of going out to a restaurant can save you a lot of money whether you follow a plant-based diet or not! Instead of dining out several times a week, eat out for an occasional treat! If you are constantly on the move and rely on fast food, begin to prepare snacks in advance. This way, you will have full control over your meals and what goes into them. Also, by staying home, this will give you a fantastic chance to work on those cooking skills!

10. Choose Whole Foods

While this may seem like a given, whole foods are going to be some of the cheapest staples you can buy! Luckily, the whole foods are going to offer the most essential nutrients as well! Some of the more popular, budget-friendly foods include brown rice, oats, potatoes, carrots, leafy greens, frozen vegetables, apples, oranges, other fruits in season, and all of the beans and lentils!

11. Think Big

Not literally, but when you buy food in bulk, you can get much more bang for your buck! When you are at the grocery store, look for the big packages or family packs. Typically, these will provide better value compared to smaller bags or containers. In this case, you will want to pay special attention to the unit price located on the price tag; this number will tell you the cost per pound. By following this rule, you can choose the cheapest option.

12. Keep it Simple, Stupid

If you are just starting the plant-based diet, there is no reason to get crazy and wild in the kitchen! Just because you are switching your diet, this does not mean that you need to become a crazy, skilled chef. Keeping your meals simple does not mean that they are going to be boring. As you can tell from the recipes earlier in this book, recipes can be easy and delicious at the same time. Often times when you use too many ingredients, this makes it tough on the pallet and your digestion tract. Do yourself a favor and start small. As you get better with this lifestyle, that is when you can experiment a bit more with your meals.

13. Buy in Season

This is vital when it comes to shopping for a plant-based diet on a budget. The good news is that food that is grown in season is cheaper and tastes much better. In the winter, keep an eye out for citrus fruits and root vegetables. In the summer, you can keep your eyes out for nectarines and watermelon. Do yourself a favor and visit your local farmers market to get the freshest produce possible. You may be surprised to learn the wide variety of food that is made available to you!

14. Frozen

Lastly, frozen fruits and vegetables. These items are typically cheaper and can be very convenient. Frozen fruits and vegetables are typically picked once they are ripe and then frozen right away; this meaning that the foods will maintain their nutrition. This is a fantastic idea, especially in the winter when fresh produce may be limited on variety and quality. Just remember to read the label of ingredients so you can avoid any added butter, sauce, or seasoning.

Meal Planning 101

While there are several hurdles you will be facing as you start a plant-based diet, one of the more popular issues is planning your meals! In the beginning, it is exciting to try out new recipes and be on point with your nutrition. Eventually, many people begin to slip up and then give up their goals of eating healthier altogether. Luckily, it doesn't have to be as complicated as people make it out to be! Instead, you can arm yourself with these meal planning tips and tricks to help you get through when you come across a tough hurdle.

The first question you may have is why should you plan your meals? As you begin a plant-based diet, you may find it to be more difficult compared to planning meals on a SAD diet. Now, you will be slightly more limited on the foods you can have during your meals. This is why you need to educate yourself on how to properly plan your plant-based meals! Planning is vital so that when you are short on time, there is less decision making.

With meal prep, you won't overthink your meals and will be prepared at any given moment.

Meal prepping is also vital to help you stick with your healthy habits. By planning ahead, you will have a lower grocery bill and be able to eat your daily nutritional needs without thinking about it on a daily basis. This is especially helpful if you are looking to lose weight! At the end of the day, you know what will work best for you. If meal prepping will help keep you accountable, it is absolutely worth the extra effort.

Before you begin the meal prepping, I suggest starting a food journal. As you cook different meals, you can start at the beginning and keep track of the foods you enjoy and the ones you don't like so much. This way, you can save time and effort when you are trying to plan meals. This can also help you stay organized with your ingredients. In the beginning, you should keep everything simple. This way, they can be batched easily and repeated in future meals.

Choosing Foods to Prep

One of the most important factors of meal prepping on a plant-based diet is the foods you are going to include on your meal plan! I want to stress that this is meant to be fun and enjoyable. Below, you will find some of my favorite tips and tricks to keep meal prep delicious and easy.

- Look for pre-cut or frozen foods; it will make your life ten times easier. Yes, it is more expensive, but you pay for convivence!
- It is okay to adjust! As you will find out, most recipes are not one taste fits all. If you feel a certain recipe is rather bland, add your own seasonings! There are no rules stating you need to stick to the recipe or else! Express your inner chef and season to your heart's desire.
- Make a list. Seriously. As you meal prep, make your grocery list as you go along. This will help you stay focused and organized when you get to the grocery store. Making a list is also a fantastic way to avoid buying foods you really shouldn't.
- Making a list is also a wonderful way to save money. This way, you will know exactly what you have at home, and nothing will go to waste. Often times, this can be a big issue with fresh produce; it doesn't have as long as a shelf-life compared to processed foods.

- Remember to add variety to your meals. Being plant-based does not mean that your meals need to be boring. There are many flavors and spices for you to try out! Experimenting is one of the best parts of a plant-based diet. You just never know what is going to spark your taste buds!

- Stick with foods you are going to enjoy. If you don't like Brussel Sprouts, don't buy them! Are they healthy? Yes. Does that mean you need to force them down your throat? No! There are plenty of options out there, keep your taste buds happy!

- Stock your kitchen with staples. There are some wonderful choices such as potatoes, lentils, quinoa, millet, beans, and rice. These are fantastic to have as you can build multiple meals around the staples. Remember that these are going to be the centerpieces of your meals from now on. Choose one and build around that ingredient and you can never go wrong with your plant-based diet.

If you are ready to commit to the lifestyle of a plant-based diet, there is no better time than the present! You have all of the information you need to help you get started; all you need to do is apply your new found knowledge of this lifestyle. Is it going to be difficult? At first, absolutely. Change can be incredibly hard, especially if you have eaten the same way your whole life. All you need to remember is that you don't have to make the changes overnight; in fact, you are encouraged to start slow! Soon enough, you will begin experiencing the health benefits, and you will wonder why you didn't start earlier. All you need to do now is believe in yourself and make that dive!

Chapter 15 Planning Your Meals

If you have been on a diet before, you may know how much time is spent thinking about what food to buy, the new recipes you have to learn, and how on earth you are going to prepare 3 full meals plus all the snacks in between. This can be a tedious task, and while trying to be helpful, a weekly food prep session where you prepare 6 meals at once can take up a significant portion of your Sunday. Intermittent fasting makes meal planning simpler by only requiring 2 or 3 meals per day—and those can be as gourmet and complex as you like, or they can be as simple as ensuring you have the 3 main macronutrients (carb, protein, fat) in a bowl. By focusing on whole, natural foods, you can make snacks as simple as an apple with some peanut butter or beautiful red pepper and some hummus. Food does not have to be complicated—it doesn't have to be the sole focus of your day, and it does not have to play such a central role in your daily life. It is there to fuel you and give you the energy to enjoy everything else that life has to offer. Intermittent fasting can simplify your life by reducing the number of decisions that you need to make about your food.

There is one meal in your day that you should pay close attention to—and whether this meal is at the traditional first-thing-in-the-morning time slot or if it's held off until noon, what you break your fast with is still the most important meal of the day. The catch is intermittent fasting is supposed to simplify your food choices, and you should aim not to obsess over your meals—but some thought does have to go into your new lifestyle.

While intermittent fasting can be a path to weight loss through calorie reduction, it isn't a starvation diet full of restrictions. One common mistake made is reducing calories unnecessarily and being obsessive about the foods they eat - or limit - once they break their fast. Your willpower is a renewable resource, but it does have a limit—and if you are restricting your timeline and being overly controlling about the calories you do consume, your willpower will reach a breaking point, and it could lead to overeating all the foods you have been so diligently avoiding, such as carbohydrates, sugars, and salty foods.

When you overeat on so-called junk food, one of the immediate repercussions is bloating from all the salt in your food; the good news is this is temporary excess water retention that can take anywhere from a few hours to a few days to pass. The real problem is overeating on high glycemic foods like baked goods, soda, white rice, pasta and bread, and unfortunately, most pizza crusts are processed white bread dough. If you don't have a meal planned to break your fast every day, you run the risk of overeating foods that will hinder your progress instead of moving you toward your goal, especially if that goal is weight loss! The trick is not taxing your willpower to its max by allowing some of your favorite foods into your day, just make sure it's not the first thing you eat to break your fast.

Keep it simple and break your fast with some steamed or sautéed vegetables; these will fill you up with a relatively small amount and will introduce nutrient-dense calories. You could also start your day with a few pieces of fruit, or if you love your daily smoothie take that as your first meal, be mindful of the content though and avoid unnecessary sugar, a simple recipe for a breakfast smoothie is 1 cup of non-dairy milk, 1 scoop of protein powder and a banana. Foods that are high in fiber, like fruits and vegetables and healthy fats like avocado and some dairy products like Greek yogurt or a good quality cheese are more likely to fill you up than other less nutrient-dense choices. Another hack is consuming all fruits, veggies, and proteins before your carbohydrates. Studies have shown that when carbohydrates are eaten last (after nutrient-dense veggies and protein), glucose levels were lower at the 30, 60- and 120-minute checks, this keeps your insulin lower for longer and leaves you to feel satiated and less likely to overeat on your next meal.

Once you have filled your stomach with high quality, nutrient-dense foods that will keep acting on your behalf, you can indulge in the simple pleasures of simple carbs - if that's what you want to do. What you resist persists so if you have cravings for sweets, or pizza, or any other so-called junk food you could enjoy a reasonable portion, if you even have room for it after all the nutrition your just ingested, but if you wait a few hours and have a slice of pizza, don't beat yourself up about it. Intermittent fasting is not a restrictive diet, it is structured but if you want to enjoy some of your favorite food just set yourself up not to overeat it by satiating your hunger with quality nutrients, be mindful of your indulgence, take a moment to savor the meal and then carry on with your happy, thriving lifestyle!

Calories — Make Them Count!

- Turmeric: This is the powerhouse of medicinally helpful spices. The key component to turmeric is a substance called curcumin, which is a powerful anti-inflammatory and antioxidant. Medicinally turmeric has been scientifically proven to suppress molecules known to cause inflammation and not only neutralize free radical but also stimulate the body to produce more of its own antioxidants. Curcumin can boost the brain hormone BDNF and can aid with improvements to brain diseases like Alzheimer's. It can also be beneficial in preventing heart disease and even helps with cancer treatments. For some of the more serious issues, you will need more than a sprinkle to your meals and can supplement with turmeric capsules which combine other ingredients to ensure it is absorbed in the bloodstream and can get to work on fighting some of the modern ages most detrimental diseases.

- Ginger: ginger root contains a component called gingerol, which is another powerful anti-inflammatory and antioxidant. One of gingers superpowers is its ability to relieve nausea and can be used to treat chemotherapy-related nausea, osteoarthritis symptoms, morning sickness, and menstrual pain. It has also been shown to be effective at improving heart disease risk factors and providing protection against age-related damage to the brain—and in elderly women, it can be used to improve brain function.

- Sage: This herb is rich in nutrients (especially vitamin K) and antioxidants as well as having antimicrobial properties which can help with oral health. It has also been shown to reduce the intensity of hot flashes and irritability brought on by menopause and can help improve brain functions to combat Alzheimer's disease.

- Fenugreek: This is an interesting herb with many potential health benefits that contain fiber and a good amount of minerals, including iron and magnesium. Studies show this herb can play a role in managing blood sugar levels and in increasing breastmilk and weight gain in newborns. It can also be used for appetite control with one study showing participants reducing their total fat intake by 17% over a 14-day period.

- Cinnamon: This sweet and popular spice contains a substance called cinnamaldehyde, which is also an antioxidant and has anti-inflammatory properties that can improve risk factors of heart disease and can lead to improvements to Alzheimer's and Parkinson's disease (in animal studies). Specifically, for fasting, cinnamon has been shown to have a potent anti-diabetic property and can reduce blood sugar levels during a fasting window.

- Cayenne pepper: This spicy spice is part of the pepper family and contains a substance called capsaicin which gives this hot pepper its medicinal properties and the well-known heat to your favorite dishes. Capsaicin has metabolism-boosting properties with the heat it brings through the process of diet-induced thermogenesis; it also brings a strong nutritional profile including antioxidants a good dose of vitamin A. Capsaicin can reduce hunger urges allowing you to maintain your fasting window more comfortably and can improve digestive health. It has also been shown to have powerful pain relief properties by suppressing a neuropeptide that carries pain signals from the body to the brain.

- Garlic: This culinary staple is incredibly nutritious, and when examined calorie for calorie, it packs a huge nutritional punch that is rich in antioxidants, manganese, Vitamin C and B6, and trace amounts of many other nutrients. High dose of garlic has been shown to be so effective at improving blood pressure that supplements can be used in place of some regular medications. Garlic has been known to protect against age-related cell damage and may reduce the risk of Alzheimer's and dementia along with common causes of chronic diseases and in some studies, it has shown an increase in estrogen production which can provide some benefits to bone health for women.

When your food can do so much, it makes sense to dust off the spice rack and incorporate some of these common kitchen ingredients to your daily life!

Conclusion

On that note, we have come to the end of this book. I want to thank you once again for choosing this book. I hope it proved to be an enjoyable and informative read and you got all the information you needed about intermittent fasting for women.

In this book, you were given all the information you need about intermittent fasting. Once you understand the way intermittent fasting works, it becomes easier to understand your body's metabolism. This diet works along with your metabolism to improve your overall health. Select a method of fasting that meets your needs and requirements. You don't have to make any drastic changes; you merely need to be mindful of when you eat. If you eat healthy and wholesome meals during the eating window, you will see an improvement in your overall health in no time.

All the recipes given in this book are easy to follow and will help cook tasty and nutritious meals. Now, all that's left is to ensure that you stock up your pantry with the necessary ingredients for cooking delicious meals. By following intermittent fasting, you can eat your way to good health and weight loss! So why don't you get started today?

Thank you and all the best!